Magnesium

Applications in Clinical Medicine

Magnesium
Applications in Clinical Medicine

Edited by
Erine A. Kupetsky, D.O.

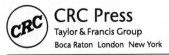

CRC Press
Taylor & Francis Group
Boca Raton London New York

CRC Press is an imprint of the
Taylor & Francis Group, an **informa** business

CRC Press
Taylor & Francis Group
6000 Broken Sound Parkway NW, Suite 300
Boca Raton, FL 33487-2742

Printed on acid-free paper

International Standard Book Number-13: 978-1-4822-2023-0 (Hardback)

Visit the Taylor & Francis Web site at
http://www.taylorandfrancis.com

and the CRC Press Web site at
http://www.crcpress.com

CV 02.01.2019 1107

Contents

About the editor

Born and raised in New York City, Dr. Erine Kupetsky completed her BA at Rutgers–NJIT and medical school at Rowan University School of Osteopathic Medicine. She completed a family medicine residency at St. Joseph's Hospital in Philadelphia, an MS in pharmacology at Thomas Jefferson University, and a dermatopharmacology fellowship at the University of Pittsburgh Medical Center. It was during her time doing research at Thomas Jefferson University that her interest in the clinical applications of magnesium in medicine began. She wanted to use her whole-patient approach to medicine and love of dermatology to help patients who had pseudoxanthoma elasticum, a disease that causes ectopic calcification and can be potentially treated with magnesium supplementation. After this research, Dr. Kupetsky completed her dermatology residency in Ohio in 2016 and worked as an employee for a large dermatology company before deciding to start her own private practice.

Contributors

Mario Barbagallo, MD
University of Palermo
Palermo, Italy

Alison Bauer, MD
Obstetrics and Gynecology
CWRU School of Medicine
Cleveland, Ohio

Jasvinder Chawla, MD
Loyola University Medical Center
    and Hines VA Hospital
Hines, Illinois

Sunny K. Chun, DO FAAD
SKC Dermatology
Fort Lee, New Jersey

Raymond Dieter, MD
Hines VA Hospital
Hines, Illinois

Robert S. Dieter, MD
Loyola University Medical Center
    and Hines VA Hospital
Maywood, Illinois

Ligia J. Dominguez
Department of Internal Medicine
    and Emergent Pathologies
University of Palermo
Palermo, Italy

Fernando Guerrero-Romero, MD
Biomedical Research Unit
Mexican Social Security Institute
Durango, Mexico

David N. Hackney, MD, MS
Maternal Fetal Medicine
University Hospitals Cleveland
    Medical Center
Cleveland, Ohio
and
Obstetrics and Gynecology
Case Western Reserve University
Cleveland, Ohio

Kiratipath Iamsakul, BS
Inventum Bioengineering
    Technologies, LLC
Chicago, Illinois

Laura Marie Jordan, DO, MS
KCU Consortium Tri-County
    Dermatology
Cuyahoga Falls, Ohio

Walter Jones, PhD
Stritch School of Medicine
Loyola University Chicago
Maywood, Illinois

Jennifer S. Kriegler, MD
Cleveland Clinic
Cleveland, Ohio

David Leehey, MD
Loyola University Medical Center
    and Hines VA Hospital
Hines, Illinois

Maria P. Martinez Cantarin, MD
Department of Medicine
Sydney Kimmel Medical College at
    Thomas Jefferson University
Philadelphia, Pennsylvania

Rebecca Michael, MD
Department of Neurology
University of California
San Francisco, California

Mark Rabbat, MD
Loyola University Medical Center
    and Hines VA Hospital
Maywood, Illinois

Elizabeth Rocha, BS
Lurie Children's Hospital
Chicago, Illinois

Martha Rodríguez-Morán, MD
Biomedical Research Unit
Mexican Social Security Institute
Durango, Mexico

Andrea Rosanoff, PhD
Center for Magnesium Education
    & Research LLC
Pahoa, Hawaii

Brian Silver, MD
UMass Memorial Medical Center/
    University of Massachusetts
    Medical School
Worcester, Massachusetts

Sanjay Singh, PhD
Hines VA Hospital
Oakbrook Terrace, Illinois

Alexandria N. Stockman, MS
Loyola University Medical Center
    and Hines VA Hospital
Maywood, Illinois

Ravi Sunderkrishnan, MD
Department of Medicine
Sidney Kimmel Medical College at
    Thomas Jefferson University
Philadelphia, Pennsylvania

James Welsh, MD
Loyola University Medical Center
    and Hines VA Hospital
Hines, Illinois

Herbert Wilde, MS, ENT
Loyola University Medical Center
    and Hines VA Hospital
Maywood, Illinois

Introduction

With myocardial infarction and stroke being the first and fifth causes of mortality in the United States, the pharmaceutical industry has been trying to produce therapies that reduce co-morbidity and mortality. Recent observational studies of magnesium have added to the list of potential therapeutic modalities that have proved useful in reducing hypertension, stroke sequelae, metabolic syndrome/dyslipidemia, and inflammatory diseases. But magnesium therapeutic modalities also have impacts in the fields of neurology, the elderly, and obstetrics.

As the U.S. population ages and lives longer, they are also exposed to multiple treatment regimens. Polypharmacia is a common problem among the geriatric population. Offering practitioners a natural, inexpensive, relatively safe option with magnesium supplementation may help control some of the common illnesses present in this population of patients while reducing their pharmaceutical burden and health-care costs. In addition, as more of the population is proactive about their health and wellness, the prevention of cardiovascular disease with magnesium supplementation needs to become a topic of conversation between health-care providers and their patients as well as the pharmaceutical industry. While case reports and small-scale observational reports on patients using magnesium are reported in the literature, a comprehensive and up-to-date text that encompasses all the therapeutic applications for magnesium is lacking.

This text will encompass the latest uses of magnesium in a clinical setting, ranging from its uses in maintaining homeostasis to its uses in the fields of dermatology, cardiology, neurology, and obstetrics. Written by contributors who are experts in their fields, it promises to be a novel, up-to-date, comprehensive collaboration of this ubiquitous dietary supplement's application in clinical medicine.

chapter one

Magnesium homeostasis

Ravi Sunderkrishnan and Maria P. Martinez Cantarin

Contents

Introduction

Magnesium is the second-most abundant intracellular cation after potassium. It is one of the four major cations handled by the kidney, the others being sodium, potassium, and calcium. It plays an important role in intracellular signaling, serving as a co-factor for enzymes involved with protein synthesis and DNA production, and maintaining membrane potential in myocytes, especially of the heart, and bone density. It is also one of the important factors involved in nerve conduction and cardiac contractility.

Total body magnesium content is 24–25 gm, 99% of which is intracellular.[1] Of these, 60% is stored predominantly in bone, in association with the apatite crystals, as a freely exchangeable divalent cation. Twenty percent of the total body magnesium concentration is localized in muscle, and the remaining 20% is distributed in other tissues. Thus, only 1% of the total body magnesium is in the extracellular fluid (ECF) compartment. Out of this, only one-third is actually present in the serum, which we usually measure. Thus, it is evident that a serum magnesium level is not reflective of the total body magnesium stores. However, our guidelines of hyper- and hypomagnesemia management are based on serum magnesium values.[2]

Dietary sources of magnesium

The nutritional recommended daily allowance (RDA) is 300 mg for women and 400 mg for men.[3] Spinach has the highest magnesium content. Other good sources of magnesium are chard, pumpkin seeds, yogurt, nuts, cocoa, avocado, black beans, and banana. Seafood like mackerel, halibut, and salmon have high magnesium levels (20% of RDA). Meats and poultry have very low levels.[4]

Refining grains and sugar and over-cooking or over-processing food cause the product to become magnesium depleted. Western diets are heavily dependent on refined flour and ready meals, so low magnesium intake is common in the United States.[5]

Measurement of magnesium and its distribution

Magnesium (Mg) exists in three different forms in the body: ionized (60%), protein bound (30%) and complexed with anions (10%).[6] Normal serum magnesium levels are 1.8–2.3 mg/dL (1.5–1.9 mEq/L). As mentioned earlier, since only one-third of the total fraction of ECF magnesium is in the serum, a serum magnesium level is an inaccurate measure of the total body magnesium. Also, the measurement of magnesium in the serum is affected by bilirubin and hemolysis.[7] Exercise and pregnancy can falsely lower serum levels. Despite these shortcomings, it is the most widely used and least cumbersome form of magnesium measurement.[8] Some authors advocate for whole-blood magnesium measurement rather than serum magnesium, as red blood cells (RBCs) contain more magnesium than the serum (1.65 to 2.65 mmol/L or 3.3 to 5.5 mEq/L). However, young RBCs and those produced due to stimulation from external erythropoietin generally have higher values, which may confound results. The muscle content of magnesium has been quantified using neutron activation analysis in laboratory experiments and in patients with Duchenne muscular dystrophy.[9] This, however, cannot be extended to everyday practice.

The fractional excretion of magnesium (FeMg) calculated in a spot urine sample is a quicker snapshot of the magnesium milieu and renal handling. In the setting of hypomagnesemia, FeMg >2% is considered renal wasting. The formula used is

$$FeMg = \frac{serum\,Cr \times urine\,Mg}{(0.7 \times serum\,Mg) \times urine\,Cr} \times 100$$

A 24-hour urine magnesium test is more accurate and still non-invasive. It depicts the renal handling of magnesium more clearly. Inappropriately high magnesium levels in the urine suggest that magnesium is being wasted by the kidneys, either as a result of nephrotoxic drugs or certain mutations. Urinary loss of <12 mg per 24 hours is considered normal. A value of >24 mg in the setting of hypomagnesemia is considered abnormal. But the accurate urine collection may prove cumbersome in some individuals.[6]

There is also the magnesium retention test, where serum and urinary magnesium values are obtained after a magnesium load. It is used to estimate magnesium malabsorption[10] and also to estimate the magnesium content of the biggest magnesium reservoir (bone).[11] Excretion of >60% of magnesium load in urine rules out magnesium depletion.

Areas of absorption

The intestine absorbs 30%–40% of ingested magnesium, but it can vary from 24% to 75% depending on the magnesium body content. A higher percentage of magnesium is absorbed in magnesium-depleted diets, and a lower percentage in areas with magnesium-rich foods. The stomach does not participate in magnesium absorption but almost the entire intestine is capable of absorbing magnesium. The absorption increases as we proceed towards the distal ileum, where one-third of the total magnesium is absorbed.[1] Extreme caution must be exercised when magnesium enemas are given in patients with chronic kidney disease, since the rectum can also absorb magnesium.[12]

The intestinal cells process magnesium both via a paracellular transport and in an active transcellular manner, similar to the nephrons. Paracellular transport depends on electrical voltage between the intestinal epithelial lumen and the blood. The active transcellular absorption takes place via transient receptor potential melastatin-6 (TRPM6), which facilitates the apical entry of the Mg+2 cation from the lumen. This transporter is present in the intestinal cells and the distal convoluted tubule (DCT).[13]

In the nephrons, the absorption of magnesium is slightly different from other ions. Eighty percent of the total plasma magnesium is filtered in the glomerulus, and most of it is absorbed downstream (up to 96% of the filtered magnesium). Unlike other ions, only 10%–20% is absorbed by the proximal convoluted tubule, most likely via paracellular pathways. Around 60%–70% of the absorption occurs in the thick ascending loop (TAL) of Henle and the remaining 10% in the DCT.

In the TAL, magnesium transport is passive via paracellular transport, and the driving force for absorption is the positive luminal transepithelial voltage. The TAL absorbs 40%–70% of the filtered magnesium. Claudin-16/paracellin-1 and claudin-19 are two tight-junction proteins that play an important role in magnesium transport via a paracellular pathway. These tight junctions' proteins are important in regulating the magnesium transport within the kidneys, based on serum magnesium levels. The TAL is also under the influence of various hormones (parathyroid hormone [PTH], calcitonin, AVP, glucagon), calcium, and other factors such as the acid base status and potassium and phosphate levels, which exert their effects on the magnesium flux. Anything that leads to the alteration of the electrochemical gradient in the tubule, as well as factors that alter the permeability of the paracellular pathways, can control magnesium transport. For example, loop diuretics lead to magnesium wasting via a loss of transepithelial voltage.

Mutations in the claudin-16/paracellin-1 gene result in familial hypomagnesemic hypercalciuric nephrocalcinosis (FHHNC)[13] and magnesium wasting. Hypomagnesemia is also a part of the presentation of Bartter and Gitelman syndromes. Mutations in the NKCC2 protein in Bartter syndrome and the NCC protein in Gitelman syndrome prevent adequate electric charge generation for the intracellular movement of magnesium. TRPM-6 channels in the DCTs participate in the ATP-dependent active transcellular absorption of magnesium. Disorders in renal TRPM-6 lead to autosomal recessive hypomagnesemia with hypocalcemia (HSH).[14]

Having named a few, the following table summarizes the major genetic mutations that result in urinary magnesium wasting (Table 1.1).

Interaction of magnesium with hormones and other ions

In vivo and in vitro observations have suggested that magnesium inhibits PTH secretion, especially in the background of low serum calcium. This is seemingly advantageous in ESRD patients who suffer from secondary hyperparathyroidism. Magnesium is reported to increase the vitamin D receptors on the parathyroid gland, as well as upregulating the FGF23 and Klotho receptor.[15] On the contrary, severe hypomagnesemia blunts PTH secretion by activating the Gα subunit of the calcium-sensing receptor (CASR).[16] Thus, PTH secretion is affected by magnesium at both higher and lower levels by varied mechanisms.

Hypomagnesemia is frequently accompanied by other electrolyte abnormalities. Hypomagnesemia with simultaneous hypokalemia is seen with loop diuretics, Bartter and Gitelman syndromes, diarrhea, and aminoglycoside toxicity. The proposed mechanism by which hypomagnesemia

Table 1.1 Genetic disorders associated with urinary magnesium wasting

Gene or protein	Disease	Symptoms	Part of nephron
Claudin 16/ paracellin-1 (*CLDN16 gene*)	Familial hypercalciuric hypocalcemia and nephrocalcinosis syndrome (FHHNC)	Hypomagnesemia, hypercalciuria, and nephrocalcinosis.	TAL
NKCC2 protein	Bartter syndrome	Hypokalemia, hyperreninemia, and hyperaldosteronism without hypertension, metabolic alkalosis, and hypercalciuria.	TAL
CASR	Autosomal dominant hypocalcemia	Hypocalcemia, low PTH, and high FeCa. More than 50% of affected patients will present with hypomagnesemia.	TAL
NCC protein	Gitleman syndrome	Hypokalemia, hyperreninemia, and hyperaldosteronism without hypertension, metabolic alkalosis, and hypocalciuria.	DCT
Rectifier type potassium channel Kir4.1(*KCNJ10* gene)	EAST/SeSAME syndrome	Epilepsy, ataxia, sensorineural deafness, and salt-wasting tubulopathy with/ without mental retardation.	DCT
Na-K ATPase gamma subunit (*FXYD2* gene)	Isolated dominant hypomagnesemia	Hypomagnesemia and hypocalciuria.	DCT
TRMP6 (*TRPM-6* gene)	HSH	Autosomal recessive hypomagnesemia with hypocalcemia.	DCT
EGF mutations	Isolated recessive hypomagnesemia	EGF is a potent TRPM6 stimulator. Thus, any receptor damage leads to hypomagnesemia via renal wasting.	DCT

(Continued)

Table 1.1 (Continued) Genetic disorders associated with urinary
magnesium wasting

Gene or protein	Disease	Symptoms	Part of nephron
Kv1.1 (*KCNA1* gene)	Isolated dominant hypomagnesemia	Muscle cramps, tetanic episodes, tremors, and muscle weakness.	DCT
Cyclin M2 (*CNNM2* gene)	Isolated dominant hypomagnesemia	Seizures, muscle weakness, vertigo, and headaches with hypomagnesemia	DCT

Note: DCT: Distal convoluted tubule; TAL: Thick ascending loop of Henle.

alters K transport is via the ROMK channel. A deficiency of intracellular
magnesium causes an alteration in the membrane potential of the ROMK
channel, causing a K+ efflux into the tubular lumen. The resultant simultaneous loss of potassium and magnesium also results in an increase in
the distal sodium (Na+) delivery and stimulates the ENaC channels, thus
maintaining the potassium loss.[17] Hence, unless magnesium is corrected,
hypokalemia will not easily improve with potassium repletion alone.

Chronic metabolic acidosis reduces the renal TRPM6 expression in
the apical membrane of the distal convoluted tubule, causing hyper-
magnesuria and thus hypomagnesemia. Conversely, chronic metabolic alkalosis causes an upregulation of TRPM6 expression, leading to
hypermagnesemia.[18]

Hypomagnesemia: Causes and treatment

Hypomagnesemia is relatively asymptomatic, and as such is underdiagnosed and undertreated. It is a common electrolyte abnormality seen in
hospitalized patients, affecting up to 65% of the critically ill patients and
15% of the general population in the hospital. Hypomagnesemia in the
ICU is associated with higher intrahospital mortality.[19,20]

Hypomagnesemia can be classified as mild (1.4–1.7 mEq/L), moderate
(1.0–1.3 mEq/L), and severe (<0.9 mEq/L). Manifestations of hypomagnesemia are varied, depending on the level. Mild-to-moderate hypomagnesemia causes mild hypokalemia and hypocalcemia and is commonly
asymptomatic, but some patients can have neuromuscular irritability,
numbness, paresthesias, weakness, or cramps. Severe drops in serum
magnesium to <1 mEq/L can lead to tetany, seizures, and arrhythmias,
especially torsades de pointes. Some patients will have positive Chvostek
and Trousseau signs on examination. Hypomagnesemia effects are exacerbated by concomitant hypocalcemia and hypokalemia.[6] The causes

of hypomagnesemia are varied, ranging from poor dietary ingestion to intestinal or renal losses.

Poor dietary ingestion

Given the ability of the intestine and kidney to maximally absorb magnesium, a lack of sufficient dietary magnesium intake is a less common cause of hypomagnesemia. Prolonged ingestion of processed, magnesium-depleted food and protein energy malnutrition can cause magnesium deficiency. Magnesium deficiency can also be seen in patients dependent on tube feedings or total parenteral nutrition, as well as alcoholics. Refeeding syndrome contributes to hypomagnesemia by virtue of triggering the hyperinsulinemic milieu that drives the magnesium intracellularly.

Intestinal magnesium loss

Malabsorption can result in hypomagnesemia. Short-gut syndrome and inflammatory bowel disease (IBD) result in intestinal losses. IBD, especially Crohn's disease, has been linked to hypomagnesemia in approximately 60% of patients. Villous atrophy and destroyed enterocytes are unable to actively absorb magnesium. Interestingly, recent studies have demonstrated that magnesium has anti-inflammatory properties. Magnesium can inhibit NF-κB phosphorylation, thus reducing the pro-inflammatory effects of TNF-α and IL-6. Thus, the loss of magnesium in Crohn's disease results in the further loss of immunomodulation.[21] Acute pancreatitis via the saponification of calcium and magnesium, intestinal resection surgeries, and diarrhea also cause malabsorption and subsequent hypomagnesemia.

The exact mechanism by which the prolonged use of proton pump inhibitors (PPIs) contributes to hypomagnesemia is unknown. PPIs may interfere with TRPM6 and TRPM7 to block active magnesium gut absorption, and also, by altering the intestinal pH, PPIs may affect the passive absorption through the H-K-ATPase and claudin channels.[22]

Renal magnesium loss

Renal loss can be divided into the categories described in Table 1.2.

Other forms of magnesium loss

Severe burns can lead to a loss of magnesium in the exudative fluid of the skin. The degree of hypomagnesemia is directly proportional to the total body surface area of the burns.[23] Also, following parathyroidectomy, there is a sequestration of magnesium from the acute mineralization of

Table 1.2 Mechanisms of renal magnesium loss

Mechanism	Disease
Increased tubular flow, resulting in gradient loss, with reduced reabsorption in the TAL	Polyuria, diabetic ketoacidosis, recovering phase of ATN, postrenal transplant, volume expansion from hyperaldosteronism or IV fluids
Renal tubular damage	Acute tubular necrosis (ATN)
Blocking the Na-K-2Cl channels with loss of transmembrane potential	Loop diuretics (direct channel inhibition), hypercalcemia (stimulation of calcium sensing receptor blocks the ROMK and Na-K-2Cl channel)
Genetic magnesium transporter mutations (refer to Table 1.1)	Bartter and Gitleman syndromes, SeSAME, FHHNC, HSH
Reduced TRPM6 expression in the tubules	Cyclosporine and tacrolimus
Reduced EGF receptor signaling, resulting in the suppression of TRPM6	Use of EGFR antagonists (e.g., cetuximab, erlotinib)
Direct renal tubular toxins, causing dose-related reversible or irreversible cellular damage	Cisplatin, aminoglycosides, amphotericin B, pentamidine, foscarnet

the osteoid bone, due to the loss of the PTH effect. This results in hungry bone syndrome, which is associated not only with hypomagnesemia but also with hypocalcemia, hypophosphatemia, and hypokalemia.[6]

Treatment of hypomagnesemia

Oral magnesium replacement is the preferred route for hypomagnesemia treatment, but intravenous magnesium sulfate (MgSO4) will be needed when patients are symptomatic. Severe magnesium deficiency in the order of 12–24 mg/kg has been described in chronic alcoholics.

No trials exist to support an optimal regimen, but the general consensus is to administer 4–6 g of intravenous (IV) MgSO4 per day for 3–5 days to replete body stores after an initial loading dose of 1–2 g over 5–60 min, depending on symptoms. One gram of IV MgSO4 contains 100 mg elemental Mg. Since plasma magnesium levels do not reflect body magnesium stores, serial FeMg assessments during treatment may help determine the duration of IV replacement. Torsades de pointes is an emergency and should be treated with 1–2 g IV magnesium sulfate over 10 min independently of plasma magnesium. For oral magnesium replacement, 240–1000 mg of elemental magnesium is provided per day, divided into two to three doses. The most common magnesium preparations are magnesium oxide (400–600 mg BID-TID for 3–4 days to start) or magnesium gluconate (can be given 500–1000 mg TID). This may, however, be limited by side effects such as diarrhea. There are preparations of magnesium chloride (Slow-Mag) that are associated with fewer GI side effects due to a sustained-release formulation and that possibly lead to better magnesium absorption. Magnesium replacement should be used cautiously in patients with renal insufficiency. Chronic kidney disease (CKD) patients should be repleted at 50%–75% of the recommended dose.

Potassium-sparing diuretics such as amiloride and triamterene block the ENaC channels, which reduces negative potential in the tubule. This increases magnesium reabsorption and may be helpful in conditions associated with persistent urinary magnesium wasting.

Hypermagnesemia: Causes and treatment

Severe hypermagnesemia is rarely encountered in clinical practice due to the excellent ability of the kidney to handle excess magnesium. The kidney is able to reduce magnesium tubular absorption from the usual 97% to almost negligible amounts in states of magnesium excess. However, conditions that decrease renal ability to excrete magnesium such as kidney disease can result in the rapid accumulation of magnesium.

The signs and symptoms of hypermagnesemia are the result of the pharmacologic effects of this ion, mainly on the nervous and cardiovascular systems. Hypermagnesemia is also associated with hypocalcemia due to the inhibition of PTH secretion. Mild hypermagnesemia (2–3 mEq/L) is normally asymptomatic. Moderate hypermagnesemia (4–6 mEq/L) can cause nausea, headaches, lethargy, and diminished deep-tendon reflexes. Deep-tendon reflexes are usually lost when blood magnesium exceeds 6 mEq/L. Severe hypermagnesemia (>6 mEq/L) can lead to respiratory paralysis, narcosis, and hypotension. Abnormal cardiac conduction may occur as blood levels of magnesium approach 10 mEq/L24. Serum levels >10 mEq/L can lead to flaccid quadriparesis, respiratory failure, and cardiac arrest.

Causes

Hypermagnesemia occurs due to reduced magnesium excretion or increase magnesium intake. Renal failure (acute and chronic) is the most common cause of hypermagnesemia due to reduced magnesium filtration and excretion. Hypermagnesemia is seen in the oliguric phase of acute renal failure, but once the renal failure starts to resolve, especially in the polyuric phase of acute tubular necrosis (ATN), the magnesium level starts to fall toward normal.

In chronic renal failure (CKD), the daily total urine excretion of magnesium falls proportionately to the degree of renal failure. In the initial stages of kidney disease (CKD stage 3) FeMg increases to overcome the loss of renal function, so plasma levels are maintained until creatinine clearance is <30 ml/min.[24]

A high intake of laxatives and antacids containing magnesium, or the use of magnesium-containing cathartics in renal failure patients, can cause hypermagnesemia. The iatrogenic administration of intravenous magnesium, especially in preeclampsia or eclampsia, can also result in hypermagnesemia. Lithium and adrenal insufficiency by unknown mechanisms have been associated with hypermagnesemia.

Treatment

In mild hypermagnesemia, discontinue all magnesium-containing salts or drugs. Immediate administration of 1 gm of IV calcium chloride or calcium gluconate can antagonize the effects of magnesium. Co-administration of loop diuretics/furosemide and saline infusion causes renal magnesium wasting. For resistant hypermagnesemia, administration of intravenous insulin (with glucose to prevent hypoglycemia) can also drive the magnesium intracellularly. For severe hypermagnesemia, hemodialysis can help remove magnesium very effectively. It is reported that magnesium losses in hemodialysis can be as high a 700 mg/session.[25] Peritoneal dialysis is slower in removing magnesium.

Conclusion

Magnesium is an important intracellular cation in the human body. Serum levels are maintained efficiently by the intestinal and renal tubular cells. Serum magnesium levels may not be an accurate snapshot of the total body magnesium. Mild changes in the levels usually go unnoticed and are asymptomatic. Magnesium interacts closely with potassium and calcium, which play a role in the manifestations and symptoms of hypo- or hypermagnesemia. It is vital to educate patients about the importance of magnesium in their diet.

References

1. Blaine J, Chonchol M, Levi M. Renal control of calcium, phosphate, and magnesium homeostasis. *Clin J Am Soc Nephrol* 2015;10:1257–72.
2. Martin KJ, Gonzalez EA, Slatopolsky E. Clinical consequences and management of hypomagnesemia. *J Am Soc Nephrol* 2009;20:2291–5.
3. Magnesium (fact sheet for health professionals). National Institute of Health: Office of Dietary Supplements. Available at https://ods.od.nih.gov/factsheets/Magnesium-HealthProfessional.
4. Marier JR. Magnesium content of the food supply in the modern-day world. *Magnesium* 1986;5:1–8.

5. Cordain L, Eaton SB, Sebastian A, et al. Origins and evolution of the Western diet: Health implications for the 21st century. *Am J Clin Nutr* 2005;81:341–54.
6. Topf JM, Murray PT. Hypomagnesemia and hypermagnesemia. *Rev Endocr Metab Disord* 2003;4:195–206.
7. Young D. *Effects of Preanalytical Variables on Clinical Laboratory Tests.* Washington, DC: AACC Press, 1997.
8. Jahnen-Dechent W, Ketteler M. Magnesium basics. *Clin Kidney J* 2012;5:i3–i14.
9. Bertorini TE, Bhattacharya SK, Palmieri GM, Chesney CM, Pifer D, Baker B. Muscle calcium and magnesium content in Duchenne muscular dystrophy. *Neurology* 1982;32:1088–92.
10. Nicar MJ, Pak CY. Oral magnesium load test for the assessment of intestinal magnesium absorption: Application in control subjects, absorptive hyper-calciuria, primary hyperparathyroidism, and hypoparathyroidism. *Miner Electrolyte Metab* 1982;8:44–51.
11. Cohen L, Laor A. Correlation between bone magnesium concentration and magnesium retention in the intravenous magnesium load test. *Magnes Res* 1990;3:271–4.
12. Tofil NM, Benner KW, Winkler MK. Fatal hypermagnesemia caused by an Epsom salt enema: A case illustration. *South Med J* 2005;98:253–6.
13. Alexander RT, Hoenderop JG, Bindels RJ. Molecular determinants of magne-sium homeostasis: Insights from human disease. *J Am Soc Nephrol* 2008;19:1451–8.
14. Schlingmann KP, Waldegger S, Konrad M, Chubanov V, Gudermann T. TRPM6 and TRPM7: Gatekeepers of human magnesium metabolism. *Biochim Biophys Acta* 2007;1772:813–21.
15. Konrad M, Schlingmann KP. Inherited disorders of renal hypomagnesae-mia. *Nephrol Dial Transplant* 2014;29 Suppl 4:iv63–iv71.
16. Quitterer U, Hoffmann M, Freichel M, Lohse MJ. Paradoxical block of para-thormone secretion is mediated by increased activity of G alpha subunits. *J Biol Chem* 2001;276:6763–9.
17. Huang CL, Kuo E. Mechanism of hypokalemia in magnesium deficiency. *J Am Soc Nephrol* 2007;18:2649–52.
18. Nijenhuis T, Renkema KY, Hoenderop JG, Bindels RJ. Acid-base status deter-mines the renal expression of Ca2+ and Mg2+ transport proteins. *J Am Soc Nephrol* 2006;17:617–26.
19. Rubeiz GJ, Thill-Baharozian M, Hardie D, Carlson RW. Association of hypomag-nesemia and mortality in acutely ill medical patients. *Crit Care Med* 1993;21:203–9.
20. Zafar MS, Wani JI, Karim R, Mir MM, Koul PA. Significance of serum mag-nesium levels in critically ill patients. *Int J Appl Basic Med Res* 2014;4:34–7.
21. Naser SA, Abdelsalam A, Thanigachalam S, Naser AS, Alcedo K. Domino effect of hypomagnesemia on the innate immunity of Crohn's disease patients. *World J Diabetes* 2014;5:527–35.
22. Perazella MA. Proton pump inhibitors and hypomagnesemia: A rare but serious complication. *Kidney Int* 2013;83:553–6.
23. Berger MM, Rothen C, Cavadini C, Chiolero RL. Exudative mineral losses after serious burns: A clue to the alterations of magnesium and phosphate metabolism. *Am J Clin Nutr* 1997;65:1473–81.
24. Cunningham J, Rodriguez M, Messa P. Magnesium in chronic kidney dis-ease stages 3 and 4 and in dialysis patients. *Clin Kidney J* 2012;5:i39–i51.
25. Massry SG, Seelig MS. Hypomagnesemia and hypermagnesemia. *Clin Nephrol* 1977;7:147–53.

chapter two

Clinical applications of magnesium in cutaneous medicine

Laura Marie Jordan and Sunny K. Chun

Contents

Introduction

This chapter will discuss potential applications of magnesium as adjunctive therapy in cutaneous conditions including pseudoxanthoma elasticum (PXE), psoriasis, hidradenitis suppurativa (HS), cutaneous lupus erythematosus, mycosis fungoides, melanoma, acne vulgaris, melasma, Hailey–Hailey disease (HHD), and atopic dermatitis.

Magnesium physiology

Magnesium is a nutritionally essential element that is necessary for many physiologic processes in humans. It is a critical factor in bone mineralization, muscle contraction, nerve impulse transmission, and a necessary co-factor for over 300 enzymes.[1] Magnesium has been shown to be relatively effective in the treatment of numerous health conditions including eclampsia, preeclampsia, arrhythmia, severe asthma, and migraine.[2] Magnesium deficiency increases the influx of calcium into cells, leading to the activation of NFκβ. Further, hypomagnesemia is associated with elevated TNFα.[3,4] Thus, hypomagnesemia results in the elevation of both NFκβ and TNFα, promoting the upregulation of pro-inflammatory cytokines.[5,6] This heightened inflammation caused by hypomagnesemia can lead to clinical disorders.[7]

Cutaneous absorption of magnesium does not occur in healthy skin under normal physiologic conditions.[7-10] Nonetheless, absorption across the normal stratum corneum is possible with high temperature or altered hydration, and absorption can take place more easily when there is damaged stratum corneum with transmembrane proteins such as SLC41A2 aiding in the intercellular transport of magnesium to other organ systems.[11]

The Dead Sea is well tolerated by bathers in part due to its magnesium-rich environment. It has been reported that the Dead Sea minerals improve skin barrier function, enhance the stratum corneum, and reduce skin roughness and inflammation.[12] The prevalent magnesium salts exhibit many favorable anti-inflammatory effects and can be used as adjunctive treatment for many inflammatory skin diseases. A study by Proksch et al. showed that after bathing subjects in a salt-rich magnesium chloride from the Dead Sea, skin hydration was enhanced and skin roughness and redness was reduced. The physiologic effects of magnesium ion salts include binding water, influencing epidermal proliferation and differentiation, and enhancing the permeability barrier.[12] Magnesium has been shown to significantly reduce the capacity of epidermal cells to activate allogenic T-cells as well as reducing the antigen-presenting cell capacity of Langerhans cells. In combination with solar radiation at the Dead Sea, the positive effects of magnesium at the skin barrier may be further enhanced. These findings support the hypothesis that the positive effects on the skin by the Dead Sea solution are due to its high magnesium content.[13]

Magnesium formulations

Magnesium has several dosage formulations pertaining to cutaneous treatment, including oral supplementation and topical variants.

Dietary supplementation

The dietary allowance of magnesium recommended by the Food and Drug Administration is up to 420 mg per day for adults. Food sources of magnesium include green leafy vegetables, legumes, whole grains, almonds, and fish. Common oral formulations of magnesium exist as magnesium oxide, magnesium hydroxide (milk of magnesia), magnesium citrate, magnesium gluconate, magnesium chloride, magnesium sulfate, magnesium lactate, and magnesium aspartate hydrochloride.[1]

Fumaric acid esters

Fumaric acid esters (FAEs) are another prospective oral supplementation of magnesium. Fumaderm is currently the only licensed FAE in Germany; it is comprised of dimethylfumarate and calcium, magnesium, and zinc salts of monoethyl hydrogen fumarate tablets.[14]

Topical therapy

Magnesium ascorbyl phosphate (MAP) is a vitamin C derivative with antioxidant effects as well as the potential to suppress skin pigmentation.[15]

Pseudoxanthoma elasticum

PXE is an inherited multi-systemic disorder that is characterized by a progressive degeneration of elastic fibers primarily in the skin, the retina, and the cardiovascular system. The classic forms of PXE are due to loss-of-function mutations in the ABCC6 gene, which encodes ABCC6, a transmembrane efflux transporter expressed primarily in the liver. Mutations in the ABCC6 gene cause the ectopic calcification and fragmentation of elastic fibers.[16]

Asymptomatic cutaneous changes are usually the first manifestation of PXE. The primary cutaneous lesions are small, yellowish papules 1–5 mm in diameter at flexural areas, such as the neck, axillae, antecubital fossae, popliteal spaces, inguinal, and periumbilical areas. As the disease progresses, the affected skin may become soft and wrinkled, hanging in redundant folds. In the retina, angioid streaks can be seen due to breaks in Bruch's membrane, the elastic-rich layer of the retina, and may be the only sign of the disease for years. Ultimately, vision impairment and, rarely, blindness may result due to consequential neovascularization, hemorrhage, and scarring. Gastrointestinal and cardiovascular complications may occur due to the calcification of the elastic media and intima of arteries. Weakened elastin in the vessel walls can cause small intestinal vessels to become fragile and bleed.[16]

Currently, there is no effective treatment available for this disorder. However, the mineral content of diet may have a significant impact on the severity of the clinical phenotype of PXE. In particular, magnesium seems to have an inhibitory effect on the mineralization of connective tissue and has been theorized to be a possible treatment for PXE.[16] The inhibitory capacity of dietary magnesium on connective tissue mineralization was confirmed in a mouse model study performed by LaRusso et al.[17]

Several recent studies suggest magnesium to be a promising first-line therapy for PXE. Kupetsky et al. reported that individuals with PXE have a statistically significant 36% increase in carotid intima-media thickness (CIMT) when compared with normotensive, age-matched, healthy patients.[18] They found a reduction of the CIMT measurements after treatment with magnesium oxide in ABCC6-/- knockout mice and concluded that CIMT may serve as a novel treatment biomarker in humans with PXE. Consistently, restricting dietary magnesium accelerates ectopic connective tissue mineralization in a mouse model of PXE (ABCC6-/-).[19,18] LaRusso et al. propose that magnesium may replace calcium in the calcium/phosphate complexes, potentially reducing the mineralization in tissues, as magnesium phosphate is more soluble than calcium phosphate.[20] LaRusso's earlier study found via micro-CT that there were no long-term adverse effects on the bone due to long-term elevated magnesium consumption.[17]

A clinical trial that incorporated magnesium demonstrated a clinical improvement of PXE patients when randomized to sevelamer hydrochloride (a phosphate binder) or placebo (both contained magnesium stearate).[21] A phase-two clinical trial completed out of the Mount Sinai School of Medicine in New York tested the efficacy of 1000 mg daily magnesium oxide supplementation on the clinical and histopathological mineralization in a cohort of patients with PXE. Researchers hypothesize that magnesium supplementation may reduce or eliminate the mineralization of elastic tissue via histological examination of the skin and ophthalmological exams. Results are pending.[22]

Psoriasis

Hypomagnesemia can also worsen other dermatologic conditions, including psoriasis. Aronson and Malick present two cases of alcohol-induced psoriasis exacerbations, which improved by adjusting their endotoxin production, low serum magnesium levels, and elevated plasma homocysteine levels.[23] Levi-Schaffer et al. researched the mechanism of the antiproliferative effect that five Dead Sea minerals had on the proliferation of fibroblasts grown from psoriatic and healthy skin specimens, investigating the potential improvement of psoriasis. The study found that the magnesium formulations had greater inhibitory effects than the potassium salts or sodium chloride and that this inhibition was present in both psoriatic and healthy skin cells.[24] Dessy et al. took this a step further by developing a topical Dead Sea mineral (DSM)-based drug delivery system by loading polymeric nanoparticles with DSMs.[25]

Moderate success has also been seen in the treatment of psoriasis with fumaric acid esters (FAEs) due to their immunomodulatory and anti-inflammatory effects. Specifically, Ghoreschi et al. found that fumarate treatment in humans interferes with the production of IL-12 and IL-23, which promote pathogenic Th-cell differentiation.[26] Psoriasis is approved to be treated with Fumaderm in Germany, an FAE containing dimethylfumarate, calcium, magnesium, and zinc salts of monoethyl hydrogen fumarate. Atwan et al.'s review of literature included six randomized controlled trials studying the FAE treatment of psoriasis and found that FAEs are more efficacious than placebo treatment and potentially equitable to methotrexate for psoriasis. However, the authors acknowledge limitations to their study, as four out of the six studies were either abstracts or reports.[27]

A rare but important side effect of FAEs is drug-induced Fanconi syndrome. Balak et al. studied 11 cases involving female patients with psoriasis with two cases displaying drug-induced Fanconi syndrome from the use of FAEs. However, the authors note that this association is rare but encourage physicians to be vigilant about monitoring for this potential side effect.[28] Reich et al. performed a retrospective data collection of 127 children and adolescents (aged 6–17 years) who were treated for up to 60 months with FAEs to treat their plaque psoriasis. The study suggests that long-term FAE treatment in this population could be effective and safe.[29]

A phase-three clinical trial completed out of the Medical University of Vienna investigated the additive effect of narrow-band type-B ultraviolet (NB-UVB) therapy in combination with FAE for the treatment of severe plaque psoriasis compared with FAE monotherapy. The study found significant improvement in PASI score with this combination therapy, indicating that adding NB-UVB improves the therapeutic response of FAEs during the early treatment of these patients.[30]

Hidradenitis suppurativa

FAE treatment of HS is also being explored. Deckers et al. tested the efficacy of FAEs on treating HS by treating seven patients with moderate to severe HS with progressive doses of FAEs up to 720 mg per day. One patient displayed evidence of improvement after 20 weeks, while two others exhibited lessened inflammation and faster-resolving lesions. After 28 weeks these three patients all displayed clear improvement, while the remaining four patients stopped after 20 weeks due to a lack of efficacy.[31]

Cutaneous lupus erythematosus

Several case reports have displayed successive treatment of cutaneous lupus erythematosus with FAEs. Tsianakas et al.'s report on the treatment of a 52-year-old woman with discoid lupus erythematosus with FAEs who experienced a decrease in discoid lesion activity and damage based on the Revised Cutaneous Lupus Disease Area and Severity Index (RCLASI).[32]

Balak and Thio present two cases of cutaneous lupus treated with FAEs: a 35-year-old woman with lupus erythematosus tumidus whose lesions reached complete resolution after 3 months of treatment with fumarates and a 24-year-old woman with systemic lupus erythematosus who was treated with combination therapy of fumarates and 10 mg prednisone, which improved her skin lesions.[33] Klein et al. present the case of a 42-year-old man with discoid lupus erythematosus who was treated with combination therapy of hydroxychloroquine and fumarates and experienced complete resolution of his erythematous lesions.[34] Although research is limited to case reports at this time, a completed phase-two clinical trial out of the University Hospital Muenster evaluated the efficacy of Fumaderm on 11 patients with cutaneous lupus erythematosus after 24 weeks of treatment. The authors found significant improvement in the clinical extent and severity of patients' lupus, indicating that FAEs could serve as alternative treatment in these patients. However, the authors did note that randomized controlled trials are still warranted.[35]

Mycosis fungoides

Magnesium ion concentration correlates with the prevalence of clinical stage mycosis fungoides (MF). Detecting low levels of magnesium and calcium have been incorporated in assessing early-stage, intermediate-stage, and advanced-stage MF. In rat studies, hypomagnesemia has been associated with immune function imbalances, leading to the development of T-cell leukemia lymphoma. A study by Morgan et al. showed that hypomagnesemia was present in 22.2% of MF patients in all stages (early, intermediate, and advanced MF), whereas hypocalcemia was present in only 8.3% of all stages. The authors hypothesize that magnesium deficiency could contribute to the development of MF or Sezary syndrome.[36] Potentially, magnesium supplementation could stave off the progression of these diseases; however, no studies to date have pursued this possibility.

Malignant melanoma

Data show that extracellular magnesium ion concentration and the rate of melanoma cell migration are directly related. Magnesium ions are known to promote integrin-mediated melanoma cell migration. In contrast, calcium ion has the opposite effect. When magnesium or calcium ions are increased in the microenvironment, there are distinct effects on melanoma cell migration on type-IV collagen. A study by Yoshinaga et al. showed that by increasing Mg^{2+} ion concentration to 5 mM yielded maximum cell migration, whereas an increase in concentration to 10 mM led to a decrease in migration. Contrary to these results, calcium levels did not lead to migration on the same substrate.[37]

Acne vulgaris

The serum levels and the roles of Zn, Cu, and Mg have been studied in acne vulgaris. Studies show that serum Mg concentration is significantly lower in severe acne groups when compared with mild acne groups. With regard to serum Cu levels, there was no significant difference between patient groups themselves or between patient and control groups.[38] Lee et al. studied the efficacy of MAP on the expression of inflammatory biomarkers in cultured sebocytes. The study found that the sebocytes treated with MAP experienced a decrease in the expression of inflammatory cytokines when compared with the sebocytes treated with lipopolysaccharide (LPS), thus concluding that MAP could potentially act as an alternative therapy to treat inflammatory acne.[39]

Melasma

Earlier studies have suggested that the topical application of magnesium formulation can reduce skin hyperpigmentation in some patients.[40] More recently, Shaikh and Mashood investigated the treatment of refractory melasma with a combination therapy of topical 5% MAP and fluorescent-pulsed light (FPL). Sixty-five patients with skin types III through V and refractory melasma received 12 weeks of treatment with topical 5% MAP and three sessions of FPL (570–950 nm) at weeks 3, 6, and 9. The patients continued to be monitored for an additional 12 weeks to evaluate the continuation of treatment benefit. The study found that the baseline mean melasma area and severity index (MASI) score of 14.80 reduced to 4.53 at the end of treatment and 6.35 at the end of follow-up. The study found that combination therapy of 5% MAP with FPL is both effective and safe in treating refractory melasma.[41]

Hailey–Hailey disease

HHD is an autosomal dominant inherited intraepidermal blistering disease caused by mutations in the ATP2C1 gene, which codes for the protein SPCA1 (secretory pathway calcium/manganese-ATPase). As a result, keratinocyte cytosolic Ca2+ concentration becomes deregulated. Borghi et al. explored the efficacy of magnesium chloride (MgCl2) in the treatment of HHD. The authors reported the significant clinical improvement of skin lesions in a patient with HHD when treated with a daily intake of MgCl2 solution. The authors investigated the effect of MgCl2 on intracellular calcium homeostasis and on the activity of calcium effectors in HeLa cells injected with chimeric aequorins. The study found that MgCl2 altered the calcium extrusor system without changing the calcium filling and releasing of stores. As such, the authors postulated that MgCl2 may act as an inhibitor of the calcium-extruding activity in keratinocytes and that this activity could explain the clinical improvement they observed in their patient.[42]

Atopic dermatitis

The evidence supporting the magnesium treatment of atopic dermatitis is fluctuating. Proksch et al. reported the improvement of skin barrier function in atopic subjects after submerging their forearms for 15 minutes in Dead Sea salt solution compared with tap water as control.[12] More recently, Heinlin et al. investigated the efficacy of synchronous balneophototherapy (narrow-band UVB treatment with synchronous bathing in Dead Sea salt solution) compared with that of narrow-band UVB therapy alone and found a statistically significant advantage in synchronous balneophototherapy after 6 months of treatment.[43] However, Togawa et al. performed a randomized, double-blind pilot study that investigated the direct effects of ultra-pure soft water, in which Ca2+ and Mg2+ have been mostly removed, on skin barrier function in child AD patients. They found that mild AD patients experienced improvement in their eczema area and severity index.[44] In a comparison study of 58 participants with hand eczema, it was found that 5% topical fumaric acid was less effective than 0.1% triamcinolone, reducing the erythema but not other eczema manifestations (excoriation, population, and lichenification).[45]

Conclusion

Magnesium has the potential to serve as an adjuvant treatment for a host of dermatologic conditions. Current studies suggest that increasing dietary magnesium as well as supplementation could prove beneficial in PXE. Additionally, magnesium deficiency could attribute to the development of MF or Sezary syndrome, so magnesium supplementation could potentially stave off the progression of these diseases.[36] However, no studies to date have pursued this possibility. A case study suggests that ingesting MgCl2 solution could improve the clinical presentation of HHD, but larger trials are needed.[42] The success of treating atopic dermatitis with magnesium is inconsistent and would benefit from larger clinical trials.

FAEs offer an exciting potential adjunctive treatment in psoriasis, HS, and cutaneous lupus erythematosus. The evidence strongly supports psoriasis treatment with FAEs, and new results are pending for a phase-three clinical trial of combination therapy with FAE and narrow-band UVB therapy. Research into the treatment of HS and FAE is in its infancy, with one small case study. Similarly, the treatment of cutaneous lupus erythematosus is also limited primarily to case studies; however, a larger 11-patient clinical trial is pending.

Magnesium ascorbyl phosphate has shown promise in the treatment of acne vulgaris and melasma. Lee et al.'s study found that sebocytes treated with MAP decreased their expression of inflammatory cytokines; however, clinical trials are needed.[39] Shaikh and Mashood found success in the treatment of refractory melasma with a combination therapy of topical 5% MAP and FPL.[41]

Research behind magnesium in the treatment of cutaneous conditions may still be in its infancy, but it is slowly growing into a burgeoning field. The prospect of magnesium treatment would greatly benefit from larger clinical trials to investigate the true depths to which its efficacy could extend.

References

1. National Institutes of Health, Office of Dietary Supplements (NIH ODS) (2013). "Magnesium fact sheets for health professionals." Retrieved January 29, 2016.
2. Guerrera, M. P., S. L. Volpe, and J. J. Mao (2009). "Therapeutic uses of magnesium." *Am Fam Physician* **80**(2): 157–162.
3. Song, Y., T. Y. Li, R. M. van Dam, J. E. Manson, and F. B. Hu (2007). "Magnesium intake and plasma concentrations of markers of systemic inflammation and endothelial dysfunction in women." *Am J Clin Nutr* **85**(4): 1068–1074.
4. Chacko, S. A., Y. Song, L. Nathan, L. Tinker, I. H. de Boer, F. Tylavsky, R. Wallace, and S. Liu (2010). "Relations of dietary magnesium intake to biomarkers of inflammation and endothelial dysfunction in an ethnically diverse cohort of postmenopausal women." *Diabetes Care* **33**(2): 304–310.
5. Weglicki, W. B., T. M. Phillips, A. M. Freedman, M. M. Cassidy, and B. F. Dickens (1992). "Magnesium-deficiency elevates circulating levels of inflammatory cytokines and endothelin." *Mol Cell Biochem* **110**(2): 169–173.
6. Malpuech-Brugère, C., E. Rock, C. Astier, W. Nowacki, A. Mazur, and Y. Rayssiguier (1998). "Exacerbated immune stress response during experimental magnesium deficiency results from abnormal cell calcium homeostasis." *Life Sci* **63**(20): 1815–1822.
7. Chandrasekaran, N. C., C. Weir, S. Alfraji, J. Grice, M. S. Roberts, and R. T. Barnard (2014). "Effects of magnesium deficiency: More than skin deep." *Exp Biol Med (Maywood)* **239**(10): 1280–1291.
8. Lansdown, A. B. (1995). "Physiological and toxicological changes in the skin resulting from the action and interaction of metal ions." *Crit Rev Toxicol* **25**(5): 397–462.
9. Hostýnek, J. J., R. S. Hinz, C. R. Lorence, M. Price, and R. H. Guy (1993). "Metals and the skin." *Crit Rev Toxicol* **23**(2): 171–235.
10. Jahnen-Dechent, W., and M. Ketteler (2012). "Magnesium basics." *Clin Kidney J* **5**(Suppl 1): i3–i14.
11. Sahni, J., B. Nelson, and A. M. Scharenberg (2007). "SLC41A2 encodes a plasma-membrane Mg2+ transporter." *Biochem J* **401**(2): 505–513.
12. Proksch, E., H. P. Nissen, M. Bremgartner, and C. Urquhart (2005). "Bathing in a magnesium-rich Dead Sea salt solution improves skin barrier function, enhances skin hydration, and reduces inflammation in atopic dry skin." *Int J Dermatol* **44**(2): 151–157.

13. Schempp, C. M., H. C. Dittmar, D. Hummler, B. Simon-Haarhaus, J. Schulte-Mönting, E. Schöpf, and J. C. Simon (2000). "Magnesium ions inhibit the antigen-presenting function of human epidermal Langerhans cells in vivo and in vitro. Involvement of ATPase, HLA-DR, B7 molecules, and cytokines." *J Invest Dermatol* **115**(4): 680–686.

14. Ngan V. (2005) "Fumaric acid esters." Retrieved January 28, 2016, from https://www.dermnetnz.org/topics/fumaric-acid-esters/.

15. Hwang, T. L., C. J. Tsai, J. L. Chen, T. T. Changchien, C. C. Wang, and C. M. Wu (2012). "Magnesium ascorbyl phosphate and coenzyme Q10 protect keratinocytes against UVA irradiation by suppressing glutathione depletion." *Mol Med Rep* **6**(2): 375–378.

16. Marconi, B., I. Bobyr, A. Campanati, E. Molinelli, V. Consales, V. Brisigotti, M. Scarpelli, S. Racchini, and A. Offidani (2015). "Pseudoxanthoma elasticum and skin: clinical manifestations, histopathology, pathomechanism, perspectives of treatment." *Intractable Rare Dis Res* **4**(3): 113–122.

17. LaRusso, J., Q. Li, Q. Jiang, and J. Uitto (2009). "Elevated dietary magnesium prevents connective tissue mineralization in a mouse model of pseudoxanthoma elasticum (Abcc6(-/-))." *J Invest Dermatol* **129**(6): 1388–1394.

18. Kupetsky, E. A., F. Rincon, and J. Uitto (2013). "Rate of change of carotid intima-media thickness with magnesium administration in Abcc6-/- mice." *Clin Transl Sci* **6**(6): 485–486.

19. Kupetsky-Rincon, E. A., Q. Li, and J. Uitto (2012). "Magnesium reduces carotid intima-media thickness in a mouse model of pseudoxanthoma elasticum: A novel treatment biomarker." *Clin Transl Sci* **5**(3): 259–264.

20. LaRusso, J., Q. Li, and J. Uitto (2011). "Pseudoxanthoma elasticum, the paradigm of heritable ectopic mineralization disorders: Can diet help?" *J Dtsch Dermatol Ges* **9**(8): 586–593.

21. Yoo, J. Y., R. R. Blum, G. K. Singer, D. K. Stern, P. O. Emanuel, W. Fuchs, R. G. Phelps, S. F. Terry, and M. G. Lebwohl (2011). "A randomized controlled trial of oral phosphate binders in the treatment of pseudoxanthoma elasticum." *J Am Acad Dermatol* **65**(2): 341–348.

22. Lebwohl, M. (2016). "Magnesium supplements in the treatment of pseudoxanthoma elasticum." Retrieved Januaray 28, 2016, from https://clinicaltrials.gov/ct2/show/NCT01525875 (Identification No. NCT02039297).

23. Aronson, P. J., and F. Malick (2010). "Towards rational treatment of severe psoriasis in alcoholics: report of two cases." *J Drugs Dermatol* **9**(4): 405–408.

24. Levi-Schaffer, F., J. Shani, Y. Politi, E. Rubinchik, and S. Brenner (1996). "Inhibition of proliferation of psoriatic and healthy fibroblasts in cell culture by selected Dead-Sea salts." *Pharmacology* **52**(5): 321–328.

25. Dessy, A., S. Kubowicz, M. Alderighi, C. Bartoli, A. M. Piras, R. Schmid, and F. Chiellini (2011). "Dead Sea minerals loaded polymeric nanoparticles." *Colloids Surf B Biointerfaces* **87**(2): 236–242.

26. Ghoreschi, K., J. Brück, C. Kellerer, C. Deng, H. Peng, O. Rothfuss, R. Z. Hussain, et al. (2011). "Fumarates improve psoriasis and multiple sclerosis by inducing type II dendritic cells." *J Exp Med* **208**(11): 2291–2303.

27. Atwan, A., J. R. Ingram, R. Abbott, M. J. Kelson, T. Pickles, A. Bauer, and V. Piguet (2015). "Oral fumaric acid esters for psoriasis." *Cochrane Database Syst Rev* **8**: CD010497.

28. Balak, D. M., J. N. Bouwes Bavinck, A. P. de Vries, J. Hartman, H. A. Neumann, R. Zietse, and H. B. Thio (2016). "Drug-induced Fanconi syndrome associated

with fumaric acid esters treatment for psoriasis: a case series." *Clin Kidney J* **9**(1): 82–89.

29. Reich, K., C. Hartl, T. Gambichler, and I. Zschocke (2016). "Retrospective data collection of psoriasis treatment with fumaric acid esters in children and adolescents in Germany (KIDS FUTURE study)." *J Dtsch Dermatol Ges* **14**(1): 50–57.

30. Tzaneva, S., A. Geroldinger, H. Trattner, and A. Tanew (2018). "Fumaric acid esters in combination with a 6-week course of narrowband ultraviolet B provides an accelerated response compared with fumaric acid esters mono-therapy in patients with moderate-to-severe plaque psoriasis: a randomized prospective clinical study." *Br J Dermatol* **178**(3): 682–688.

31. Deckers, I. E., H. H. van der Zee, D. M. Balak, and E. P. Prens (2015). "Fumarates, a new treatment option for therapy-resistant hidradenitis sup-purativa: A prospective open-label pilot study." *Br J Dermatol* **172**(3): 828–829.

32. Tsianakas, A., S. Herzog, A. Landmann, N. Patsinakidis, A. M. Perusquía Ortiz, G. Bonsmann, T. A. Luger, and A. Kuhn (2014). "Successful treat-ment of discoid lupus erythematosus with fumaric acid esters." *J Am Acad Dermatol* **71**(1): e15–e17.

33. Balak, D., and H. Thio (2011). Treatment of lupus erythematosus with fumaric acid esters: Two case-reports. *J Transl Med.* **9**.

34. Klein, A., B. Coras, M. Landthaler, and P. Babilas (2012). "Off-label use of fumarate therapy for granulomatous and inflammatory skin diseases other than psoriasis vulgaris: A retrospective study." *J Eur Acad Dermatol Venereol* **26**(11): 1400–1406.

35. Kuhn, A., A. Landmann, N. Patsinakidis, V. Ruland, S. Nozinic, A. M. Perusquía Ortiz, C. Sauerland, T. Luger, A. Tsianakas, and G. Bonsmann (2016). "Fumaric acid ester treatment in cutaneous lupus erythematosus (CLE): a prospective, open-label, phase II pilot study." *Lupus* **25**(12):1357–1364.

36. Morgan, M., D. Maloney, and M. Duvic (2002). "Hypomagnesemia and hypo-calcemia in mycosis fungoides: A retrospective case series." *Leuk Lymphoma* **43**(6): 1297–1302.

37. Yoshinaga, I. G., S. K. Dekker, M. C. Mihm, and H. R. Byers (1994). "Differential effect of magnesium and calcium on integrin-mediated mela-noma cell migration on type IV collagen and fibronectin." *Melanoma Res* **4**(6): 371–378.

38. Saleh, B., Z. Anbar, and A. Majid (2013). Role of some trace elements in pathogenesis and severity of acne vulgaris in Iraqi male patients. *J Clin Exp Dermatol Res.*

39. Lee, W. J., S. L. Kim, Y. S. Choe, Y. H. Jang, S. J. Lee, and D. W. Kim (2015). "Magnesium ascorbyl phosphate regulates the expression of inflammatory biomarkers in cultured sebocytes." *Ann Dermatol* **27**(4): 376–382.

40. Kameyama, K., C. Sakai, S. Kondoh, K. Yonemoto, S. Nishiyama, M. Tagawa, T. Murata, et al. (1996). "Inhibitory effect of magnesium L-ascorbyl-2-phosphate (VC-PMG) on melanogenesis in vitro and in vivo." *J Am Acad Dermatol* **34**(1): 29–33.

41. Shaikh, Z. I., and A. A. Mashood (2014). "Treatment of refractory melasma with combination of topical 5% magnesium ascorbyl phosphate and fluores-cent pulsed light in Asian patients." *Int J Dermatol* **53**(1): 93–99.

42. Borghi, A., A. Rimessi, S. Minghetti, M. Corazza, P. Pinton, and A. Virgili (2015). "Efficacy of magnesium chloride in the treatment of Hailey–Hailey

disease: From serendipity to evidence of its effect on intracellular Ca(2+) homeostasis." *Int J Dermatol* **54**(5): 543–548.

43. Heinlin, J., J. Schiffner-Rohe, R. Schiffner, B. Einsele-Krämer, M. Landthaler, A. Klein, F. Zeman, W. Stolz, and S. Karrer (2011). "A first prospective randomized controlled trial on the efficacy and safety of synchronous balneophototherapy vs narrow-band UVB monotherapy for atopic dermatitis." *J Eur Acad Dermatol Venereol* **25**(7): 765–773.

44. Togawa, Y., N. Kambe, N. Shimojo, T. Nakano, Y. Sato, H. Mochizuki, A. Tanaka, H. Matsuda, and H. Matsue (2014). "Ultra-pure soft water improves skin barrier function in children with atopicss dermatitis: a randomized, double-blind, placebo-controlled, crossover pilot study." *J Dermatol Sci* **76**(3): 269–271.

45. Jowkar, F., N. Saki, A. Mokhtarpour, and M. R. Saki (2014). "Comparison of fumaric acid 5% cream versus triamcinolone 0.1% cream in the treatment of hand eczema." *Acta Med Iran* **52**(7): 528–531.

chapter three

Magnesium in the elderly

Mario Barbagallo and Ligia J. Dominguez

Contents

Introduction

Aging is frequently associated with a clinical or subclinical magnesium (Mg) deficit. Several alterations to Mg status have been identified in the elderly.[1–13] Total body Mg content (1000–1100 mmol) tends to decrease with age. Bone is the main storage compartment of the body's Mg. About 55%–65% of the total Mg content is stored in the mineral phase of the skeleton, 34%–44% in the intracellular space, and only 1% in the extracellular fluid.[14] Although Mg content in bone is not easily exchanged, the age-related reduction of bone mass that occurs both in men and women is associated with a reduction of total body minerals and Mg content (Figure 3.1).

The equilibrium of Mg homeostasis and the Mg concentrations in plasma and in the cells are tightly regulated,[14–17] and changes in plasma Mg can occur only in the presence of a significantly long-lasting Mg depletion. Although no known hormonal factor is specifically involved in the regulation of Mg metabolism, many hormones are known to affect Mg balance and transport, such as parathyroid hormone (PTH), calcitonin, vitamin D, catecholamines, and insulin. In particular, there is an important link between Mg and calciotropic hormones, since not only PTH and vitamin D may regulate Mg homeostasis, but Mg itself is essential for the normal function of the parathyroid glands, for vitamin D metabolism, and to ensure the adequate sensitivity of target tissues to PTH and active vitamin D metabolites.[18,19] It is thus likely that the modification of these

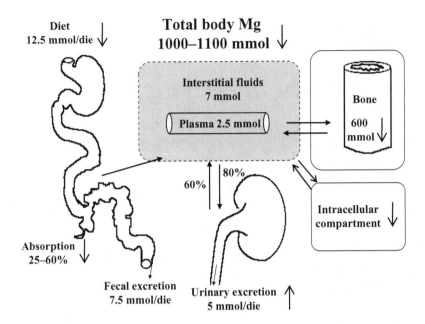

Figure 3.1 Mg homeostasis with age.

regulating hormones with age (decreased vitamin D status and increased PTH levels)[20,21] may affect Mg homeostasis in the elderly, although these aspects have not been completely elucidated.

Total plasma Mg concentrations (MgT), also in relation to this tight control, are remarkably constant in healthy subjects throughout life and do not tend to change with aging[1,6] (Figure 3.2a). MgT is in large part bound to proteins or chelated, and it is not very sensitive in detecting subclinical Mg deficiencies. Possible changes may depend mainly on

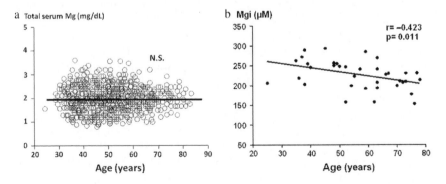

Figure 3.2 Relationship of (a) total serum Mg and (b) intracellular free Mg (Mgi) to aging.

age-related diseases, therapies, and age-related changes in renal function. Twenty-four-hour Mg retention studies have revealed an increased Mg retention in the elderly, suggesting a significant subclinical Mg deficit, not easily detected by total serum Mg.[10] The use of a Mg ion-selective electrode (ISE) to measure the active ionized free Mg (Mg-ion) has been suggested for the detection of some of these subclinical Mg deficits. A close direct relationship was found between Mg-ion and the intracellular Mg measurement.[22] In clinical practice, the measurement of the active ionized free Mg in the serum may allow a higher sensitivity than MgT in detecting subclinical Mg deficits in several clinical conditions, including aging. In preliminary data in healthy adults aged over 65 years, we have found a slight but significant reduction in Mg-ion compared to younger controls, changes which were not detected by the measurement of total serum Mg (Table 3.1).

Mg in the intracellular compartment also tends to reduce with aging. Intracellular free Mg has been found to be significantly decreased in healthy persons aged over 65 years compared with younger (<65 years) controls.[11,12] We have specifically studied the behavior of intracellular Mg content with age, using ^{31}P-nuclear magnetic resonance (NMR) spectroscopy in peripheral red blood cells from healthy adults and have shown a continuous age-dependent fall of intracellular Mg levels in healthy elderly subjects,[12] without significant changes in total serum Mg (Figure 3.2b). Thus, at least in conditions associated with a subclinical Mg deficit, the compartments that seem to be initially compromised are the intracellular compartments and the ionized fraction of serum Mg, while a reduction of the bound and complexed total serum Mg (hypomagnesemia) may appear only at a later stage in relation to more considerable and longer-lasting Mg depletion.

Mechanisms of Mg deficits with age

The most common mechanisms linked to Mg deficits with aging are summarized in Table 3.2. A decreased intake of Mg has been suggested to play a primary role in age-related Mg deficit. Epidemiological studies have shown that Mg intake in western countries tends to decrease with aging.[23–28]

Table 3.1 Ionized and total magnesium in the elderly (aged ≥65 years) versus young (aged <65 years) persons

Group	Mg Tot (mg/dL)	Mg Ion (mmol/L)
Young (aged <65 years)	2.0 ± 0.5	0.521 ± 0.01
Old (aged ≥65 years)	1.9 ± 0.5	0.496 ± 0.02*

*$p < 0.001$ vs. young subjects.

Table 3.2 Mechanisms of magnesium deficits with aging

- Inadequate Mg nutrient intake
- Reduced efficiency of Mg absorption (associated with reduced vitamin D levels)
- Increased Mg urinary excretion (associated with age-dependent reduction of kidney function and Mg tubular reabsorption)
- Secondary Mg deficiency (associated with diseases and comorbidities, and/ or increased urinary Mg loss linked to polypharmacy)

This is probably because the elderly tend to consume more processed foods with low content in whole grains and green vegetables. Although it has been shown that Mg requirements do not change with age,[28] dietary Mg deficiency in the elderly is more prevalent than generally suspected. Data from the National Health and Nutrition Examination Survey (NHANES) III found that Mg daily intake progressively decreases with age,[23] and that those affected by chronic conditions and/or on chronic drug treatment are less likely than younger adults to consume enough Mg to meet their needs. The NHANES III survey has confirmed that Mg intake in the older population is below the recommended minimal quantity (average of 225 and 166 mg/day vs. recommended 420 and 320 mg/day for men and women, respectively).[23] Among U.S. adults, 68% consume less than the recommended daily allowance (RDA) of Mg, 45% consume less than 75% of the RDA, and 19% consume less than 50% of the RDA.[29] In Europe, the "Suppléments en Vitamines et Minéraux Antioxidants" (SU.VI.MAX) study showed that 77% of women and 72% of men have dietary Mg intakes lower than the RDA; 23% of women and 18% of men consumed less than two-thirds of the RDA.[24] In addition to the inadequate nutrient intake, other possible pathogenetic factors that may contribute to a Mg depletion with age include a decreased Mg absorption and/or an increased urinary Mg loss, as well as multiple drug use.

The efficiency of Mg absorption declines with age. Mg is absorbed by both passive and active processes mostly in the duodenum and in the ileum. A reduction of the absorption of Mg from the intestine in the elderly may be influenced by the reduction of vitamin D metabolism with age.[1–3]

Renal active reabsorption of Mg takes place in the loop of Henle, in the proximal convoluted tubule, and is influenced by both, the urinary concentration of sodium, and urinary pH. An increased renal Mg excretion may also contribute to the Mg deficit and is linked to a reduced tubular reabsorption associated with a reduced renal function, which is a common condition in the elderly. Drug use (i.e., long-term treatment with loop diuretics, digitalis) and/or pathological conditions associated with aging (i.e., type 2 diabetes mellitus, hyperadrenoglucocorticism, insulin resistance, alcoholism, acute myocardial infarction, stroke, among others) are also associated with secondary Mg deficiencies.[2,3,5,6]

Aging, Mg, and inflammation

Aging is associated with increased oxidative stress and with a chronic, low-grade inflammation, a term coined "inflamm-aging,"[30] which has been implicated as a predictor or contributor to several chronic diseases and conditions associated with aging, including cardiovascular disease, osteoarthritis, osteoporosis, Alzheimer's disease, insulin resistance, diabetes, muscle wasting, and frailty.[30] Although the literature provides evidence connecting inflammation or inflammatory mediators and aging and with chronic diseases, most studies are correlative, while the underlying biology connecting the mediators of inflammation with these various disease processes is unclear. Because the direct effects of aging on inflammatory responses and disease pathophysiology are poorly understood, it is not surprising that a direct causal role of inflammation in age-related diseases has yet to be demonstrated. Some studies suggest a possible role of Mg in this age-related activation of low-grade inflammation.[31,32] In fact, hypomagnesemia has been associated with inflammation and the increased production of free oxygen radicals. Poor Mg status may trigger the development of a pro-inflammatory state both by causing the excessive production and release of interleukin (IL)-1β and tumor necrosis factor (TNF)-α and by elevating circulating concentrations of pro-inflammatory neuropeptides that trigger the activation of low-grade chronic inflammation.[31,32] In experimental animals, several studies have shown that Mg deprivation causes the marked elevation of pro-inflammatory molecules TNF-α, IL-1β, IL-6, vascular cell adhesion molecule (VCAM)-1, plasminogen activator inhibitor (PAI)-1, increased circulating inflammatory cells, and increased hepatic production and release of acute phase proteins (i.e., complement, α2-macroblobulin, fibrinogen).[32–39] Experimental studies in rats have shown that Mg deficiency induces the chronic impairment of redox status associated with inflammation, which could contribute to increased oxidized lipids and may promote hypertension and vascular disorders.[35]

In humans, clinical data have shown that low serum Mg levels as well as inadequate dietary Mg are strongly related to low-grade systemic inflammation.[29,40,41] Data from the Women's Health Study have shown that Mg intake is inversely associated with systemic inflammation, measured by serum C-reactive protein (CRP) concentrations, and with the prevalence of the metabolic syndrome in adult women.[36] Using the 1999–2002 NHANES database, King et al. found that dietary Mg intake was inversely related to CRP levels. Among the 70% of the population not taking supplements, Mg intake below the RDA was significantly associated with a higher risk of having elevated CRP.[29] Several other studies have confirmed an inverse relationship among Mg intake, serum Mg and TNF-α, IL-6, and CRP levels.[42–44] In a cross-sectional study, a higher TNF-α concentration was inversely associated with serum Mg and in a multivariate analysis, those with the lowest serum Mg were 80% more likely to have higher circulating levels of TNF-α.[44]

Mg deficiency has been associated, both in experimental animal models and in humans, with increased oxidative stress and decreased antioxidant defense due, at least in part, to increased inflammation parameters.[37,45,46] Previous studies have shown convincingly that Mg deficiency results in the increased production of oxygen-derived free radicals in various tissues, increased free-radical-elicited oxidative tissue damage, the increased production of superoxide anion by inflammatory cells, decreased antioxidant enzyme expression and activity, decreased cellular and tissue antioxidant levels, and increased oxygen peroxide production.[2,35,47,48] Mg may also prevent oxygen radical formation by scavenging free radicals and by inhibiting xanthine oxidase and nicotinamide adenine dinucleotide phosphate (NADPH) oxidase.[49] There is also evidence showing that Mg plays a role in the immune response as a co-factor for immunoglobulin (Ig) synthesis, C3 convertase, immune cell adherence, antibody-dependent cytolysis, IgM lymphocyte binding, macrophage response to lymphokines, and T helper-β cell adherence.[50,51]

Mg and age-related cardiovascular and metabolic diseases

Mg deficit in elderly people may cause increased vulnerability to several age-related diseases. The role of Mg in the regulation of cellular glucose metabolism and insulin action and sensitivity, as well as in the modulation of vascular smooth muscle tone and blood pressure homeostasis is well established.[12,14,52,53] Chronic Mg deficits have been linked to an increased risk of cardiovascular and metabolic diseases, including hypertension, stroke, atherosclerosis, ischemic heart disease, cardiac arrhythmias, glucose intolerance, insulin resistance, type 2 diabetes mellitus, endothelial dysfunction, vascular remodeling, alterations in lipid metabolism, platelet aggregation/thrombosis, inflammation, oxidative stress, cardiovascular mortality, asthma, and chronic fatigue, as well as depression and other neuropsychiatric disorders,[54–60] all conditions mostly observed in the elderly population.

At the cellular level, cytosolic free Mg levels (Mgi) are consistently reduced in subjects with type 2 diabetes mellitus. Using gold-standard NMR techniques, our group has shown significantly lower steady-state Mgi and reciprocally increased cytosolic free calcium levels (Cai) in subjects with type 2 diabetes, compared with young nondiabetic subjects.[12,61] Mgi depletion in diabetes has been shown to be clinically and pathophysiologically significant, since Mgi levels quantitatively and inversely predict the fasting and post-glucose levels of hyperinsulinemia, as well as peripheral insulin sensitivity, and both systolic and diastolic blood pressure.[12,14,52,53,61]

In a study of elderly patients with type 2 diabetes, we observed that ionized and Mg-T circulating levels were significantly lower in diabetic persons compared with nondiabetic controls. After adjusting for relevant confounders, Mg-tot was significantly associated with fasting blood glucose in all the participants, while ionized Mg was significantly associated with both fasting blood glucose and with HbA1c in diabetic participants.[62]

In diabetic subjects, both low Mg intake and increased Mg urinary losses have been associated with Mg deficits.[52,53] Hyperglycemia and hyperinsulinemia may both have a role in the increased urinary Mg excretion contributing to Mg depletion. A depletion of Mg seems to be a co-factor in the further derangement of insulin resistance. A Mg-deficient diet has been associated with the significant impairment of insulin-mediated glucose uptake and with an increased risk of developing glucose intolerance and diabetes.[63] Epidemiologic data have shown a significant inverse association between Mg intake and diabetes risk.[41,63] A deficient Mg status may both be a secondary consequence or precede and cause insulin resistance and altered glucose tolerance, and even diabetes.[60,64-67]

Inflammation and oxidative stress may be a link between Mg deficit and insulin resistance/metabolic syndrome.[42-44] More generally, chronic hypomagnesemia and conditions commonly associated with Mg deficiency, such as type 2 diabetes and aging, are all associated with an increase in free radical formation with subsequent damage to cellular processes.[1,2,42-44] Antioxidant therapies with vitamin E and glutathione may improve insulin sensitivity and whole body glucose disposal, and their action may be, at least in part, mediated by the effect to improve cellular Mg homeostasis.[68-70]

Altogether, these data are consistent with the role of Mg deficiency in promoting oxidative stress, inflammation, insulin resistance, vascular remodeling, atherosclerosis, type 2 diabetes, and cardiometabolic syndrome.

Mg and age-related sarcopenia

Older age is frequently characterized by a loss of skeletal muscle mass and function (sarcopenia).[71] Mg depletion may have a role in this phenomenon, causing muscle cell alterations through increased oxidative stress and impaired intracellular calcium homeostasis.[72] Thus, it has been suggested that Mg status may affect muscle performance, probably due to Mg's key role in energetic metabolism, transmembrane transport, and muscle contraction and relaxation.[14,15]

Mg supplementation (up to 8 mg/kg daily) enhanced muscle strength in young untrained individuals.[73] Similarly, physically active young persons experienced improved endurance performance and decreased oxygen use during submaximal exercise after Mg supplementation.[74] Sarcopenic older adults have a lower intake of Mg compared with nonsarcopenic older controls.[75]

Using data from the InCHIANTI study, a well-characterized representative sample of older men and women, we observed a significant, independent, and strong relationship between circulating Mg and muscle performance, which was consistent across several muscle parameters for both men and women.[76] This data is consistent (1) with the link between Mg status and muscle ATP and with the role of Mg in energetic metabolism, (2) with the increased reactive oxygen species (ROS) production in Mg deficiency, and (3) with the pro-inflammatory effect of Mg depletion. Oral Mg supplementation improved physical performance in healthy elderly women.[77]

Mg and the aging process

Mg is an essential co-factor in cell proliferation and differentiation and in all steps of nucleotide excision repair and is involved in base excision repair and mismatch repair.[78–80] DNA is continuously damaged by environmental mutagens and by endogenous processes. Mg is required for the removal of DNA damage generated by environmental mutagens, endogenous processes, and DNA replication.[78,79,81] In cellular systems, Mg, at physiologically relevant concentrations, is required to maintain genomic stability. Mg has stabilizing effects on DNA and chromatin structure, and it is an essential co-factor in almost all enzymatic systems involved in DNA processing.[78] Intracellular free Mg is a "second messenger" for downstream events in apoptosis. Thus, the levels of intracellular free Mg increase in cells undergoing apoptosis. This increase is an early event in apoptosis, preceding DNA fragmentation and the externalization of phosphatidylserine, and is likely due to a mobilization of Mg from the mitochondria.[80] There is increasing evidence from animal experiments and epidemiological studies that Mg deficiency may decrease membrane integrity and membrane function, increasing the susceptibility to oxidative stress, cardiovascular heart diseases, as well as accelerated aging, as follows. Several studies have reported alterations in cell physiology with senescence features during Mg deficiency in different cell types. Mg-related alterations may include reduced oxidative stress defense, cell cycle progression, culture growth, and cellular viability,[33,48,80,82,83] as well as the activation of the expression of proto-oncogene (e.g., c-fos, c-jun) and of transcription factors (e.g., NF-K B).[84] Mg deficiency may accelerate cellular senescence in cultured human fibroblasts.[85] Continuous cultures of primary fibroblasts in Mg-deficient media resulted in a loss of replicative capacity with accelerated expression of senescence-associated biomarkers. A marked decrease in the replicative lifespan was seen compared with fibroblast populations cultured in standard Mg media conditions. Human fibroblast populations cultured in Mg-deficient conditions also showed an increased senescence-associated β-galactosidase activity. Activation of cellular aging (p53 and pRb) pathways by Mg-deficient conditions also increased the expression of proteins associated with cellular senescence. Telomere attrition was found to be accelerated in cell populations from Mg-deficient cultures, suggesting that the long-term consequence of inadequate Mg availability in human fibroblast cultures was accelerated cellular senescence.[85]

Conclusions

An adequate Mg content is a critical factor for normal cellular and body homeostasis. Aging is very often associated with Mg status inadequacy. Chronic Mg deficiency is associated with inflammation and oxidative stress, as well as with an increased incidence of chronic diseases associated with aging. A chronic, low-grade inflammation and increased oxidative stress are underlying conditions present in many age-related diseases and have been proposed to be involved in the aging process itself. We suggest that the chronic Mg deficit may be at least one missing link activating the inflammatory process during aging and connecting inflammation with the aging process and many age-related diseases (Figure 3.3). The possibility that maintaining an optimal Mg balance throughout life

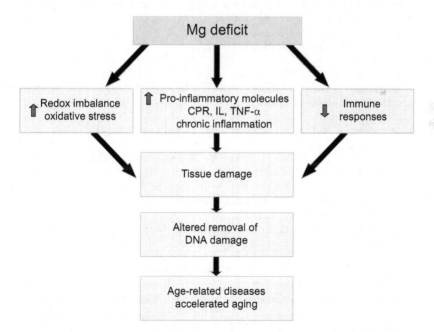

Figure 3.3 Overall hypothesis in which chronic Mg deficit has been proposed as one of the physiopathological links that may help to explain the interactions among inflammation, oxidative stress, and altered immune responses with the aging process and age-related diseases.

might help in preventing or significantly retarding the inflammation process and the manifestations of chronic diseases needs to be proven by prospective studies.

References

1. Barbagallo M, Dominguez LJ. Magnesium and aging. *Curr Pharm Des* 2010; 16:832–9.
2. Rayssiguier Y, Durlach J, Gueux E, Rock E, Mazur A. Magnesium and aging: 1. Experimental data: importance of oxidative damage. *Magnes Res* 1993; 6:373–82.
3. Davidovic M, Trailov D, Milosevic D, Radosavljevic B, Milanovic P, Djurica S, et al. Magnesium, aging, and the elderly patient. *ScientificWorldJournal* 2004; 4:544–50.
4. Lo CS, De Gasperi RN, Ring GC. Aging and whole body electrolytes in inbred A crossed with C rats. *Gerontologia* 1968; 14:1–14.
5. Sherwood RA, Aryanagagam P, Rocks BF, Mandikar GD. Hypomagnesium in the elderly. *Gerontology* 1986; 32:105–9.
6. Yang XY, Hossein JM, Ruddel ME, Elin RJ. Blood magnesium parameters do not differ with age. *J Am Coll Nutr* 1990; 9:308–13.
7. Petersen B, Schroll M, Christiansen C, Transbol I. Serum and erythrocyte magnesium in normal elderly Danish people: Relationship to blood pressure and serum lipids. *Acta Med Scand* 1977; 201:31–4.
8. McLelland AS. Hypomagnesemia in elderly hospital admissions: A study of clinical significance. *Q J Med* 1991; 78:177–84.
9. Cohen L, Kitzes R. Characterization of the magnesium status of elderly people by the Mg tolerance test. *Magnes Bull* 1992; 14:133–4.
10. Gullestad L, Nes M, Rønneberg R, Midtvedt K, Falch D, Kjekshus J. Magnesium status in healthy free-living elderly Norwegians. *J Am Coll Nutr* 1994; 13:45–50.
11. Tsunematsu K, Tanuma S, Sakuma Y. Lymphocyte Mg values in Japanese determined by microanalysing methods. *J Jpn Soc Magnes Res* 1987; 6:33–43.
12. Barbagallo M, Gupta RK, Dominguez LJ, Resnick LM. Cellular ionic alterations with age: relation to hypertension and diabetes. *J Am Geriatr Soc* 2000; 48: 1111–6.
13. Ford ES, Mokdad AH. Dietary magnesium intake in a national sample of US adults. *J Nutr* 2003; 133:2879–82.
14. Barbagallo M, Dominguez LJ. Magnesium metabolism in type 2 diabetes mellitus, metabolic syndrome and insulin resistance. *Arch Biochem Biophys* 2007; 458:40–7.
15. Wolf FI, Cittadini A. Chemistry and biochemistry of magnesium. *Mol Aspects Med* 2003; 24:3–9.
16. Saris NE, Mervaala E, Karppanen H, Khawaja JA, Lewenstam A. Magnesium: An update on physiological, clinical and analytical aspects. *Clin Chim Acta* 2000; 294:1–26.
17. Rude RK, Singer FR. Magnesium deficiency and excess. *Annu Rev Med* 1981; 32:245–59.
18. Zofková I, Kancheva RL. The relationship between magnesium and calciotropic hormones. *Magnes Res* 1995; 8:77–84.

19. Iwasaki Y, Asai M, Yoshida M, Oiso Y, Hashimoto K. Impaired parathyroid hormone response to hypocalcemic stimuli in a patient with hypomagnesemic hypocalcemia. *J Endocrinol Invest* 2007; 30:513–6.

20. Baker MR, Peacock M, Nordin BE. The decline in vitamin D status with age. *Age Ageing* 1980; 4:249–52.

21. Gallagher JC, Riggs BL, Jerpbak CM, Arnaud CD. The effect of age on serum immunoreactive parathyroid hormone in normal and osteoporotic women. *J Lab Clin Med* 1980; 95:373–85.

22. Resnick LM, Altura BT, Gupta RK, et al. Intracellular and extracellular magnesium depletion in type II (non-insulin-dependent) diabetes mellitus. *Diabetologia* 1993; 36:767–70.

23. Ford ES, Mokdad AH. Dietary magnesium intake in a national sample of US adults. *J Nutr* 2003; 133:2879–82.

24. Galan P, Preziosi P, Durlach V, et al. Dietary magnesium intake in a French adult population. *Magnes Res* 1997; 10:321–8.

25. Vaquero MP. Magnesium and trace elements in the elderly: Intake, status and recommendations. *J Nutr Health Aging* 2002; 6:147–53.

26. Berner YN, Stern F, Polyak Z, Dror Y. Dietary intake analysis in institutionalized elderly: A focus on nutrient density. *J Nutr Health Aging* 2002; 6:237–42.

27. Padro L, Benacer R, Foix S, Maestre E, Murillo S, Sanviçens E, et al. Assessment of dietary adequacy for an elderly population based on a Mediterranean model. *J Nutr Health Aging* 2002; 6:31–3.

28. Hunt CD, Johnsom LK. Magnesium requirements: new estimations for men and women by cross-sectional statistical analyses of metabolic magnesium balance data. *Am J Clin Nutr* 2006; 84:843–52.

29. King DE, Mainous AG, 3rd, Geesey ME, Woolson RF. Dietary magnesium and C-reactive protein levels. *J Am Coll Nutr* 2005; 24:166–71.

30. Franceschi C, et al. Inflamm-aging: An evolutionary perspective on immunosenescence *Ann NY Acad Sci* 2000; 908:879–96.

31. Weglicki WB, Dickens BF, Wagner TL, Chemielinska JJ, Phillips TM. Immunoregulation by neuropeptides in magnesium deficiency: Ex vivo effect of enhanced substance P production on circulation T lymphocytes from magnesium-deficient mice. *Magnes Res* 1996; 9:3–11.

32. Kramer JH, Mak IT, Phillips TM, Weglicki WB. Dietary magnesium intake influences circulating pro-inflammatory neuropeptide levels and loss of myocardial tolerance to postischemic stress. *Exp Biol Med* 2003; 228:665–73.

33. Maier JAM, Malpuech-Brugère C, Zimowska W, Rayssiguier Y, Mazur A. Low magnesium promotes endothelial cell dysfunction: Implications for atherosclerosis, inflammation and thrombosis. *Biochim Biophys Acta* 2004; 1689:13–21.

34. Bernardini D, Nasulewicz A, Mazur A, Maier JAM. Magnesium and microvascular endothelial cells: A role in inflammation and angiogenesis. *Front Biosci* 2005; 10:1177–82.

35. Blache D, Devaux S, Joubert O, Loreau N, Schneider M, Durand P, et al. Long-term moderate magnesium-deficient diet shows relationships between blood pressure, inflammation and oxidant stress defense in aging rats. *Free Rad Biol Med* 2006; 41:277–84.

36. Malpuech-Brugere C, Nowacki W, Daveau M, Gueux E, Linard E, Rock C, et al. Inflammatory response following acute magnesium deficiency in the rat. *Biochim Biophys Acta* 2000; 1501:91–8.

37. Weglicki WB, Phillips TM. Pathobiology of magnesium deficiency: A cyto-kine/neurogenic inflammation hypothesis. *Am J Physiol* 1992; 263:R734–7.
38. Kurantsin-Mills J, Cassidy MM, Stafford RE, Weglicki WB. Marked altera-tions in circulating inflammatory cells during cardiomyopathy develop-ment in a magnesium-deficient rat model. *Br J Nutr* 1997; 78:845–55.
39. Bussiere FI, Tridon A, Zimowska W, Mazur A, Rayssiguier Y. Increase in complement component C3 is an early response to experimental magne-sium deficiency in rats. *Life Sci* 2003; 73:499–507.
40. Guerrero-Romero F, Rodríguez-Morán M. Relationship between serum magnesium levels and C-reactive protein concentration in non-diabetic, non-hypertensive obese subjects. *Int J Obes Relat Metab Disord* 2002; 26:469–74.
41. Song Y, Ridker PM, Manson JE, Cook NR, Buring JE, Liu S. Magnesium intake, C-reactive protein, and the prevalence of metabolic syndrome in middle-aged and older U.S. women, *Diabetes Care* 2005; 28:1438–44.
42. King DE, Mainous AG, 3rd, Geesey ME, Ellis T. Magnesium intake and serum C-reactive protein levels in children. *Magnes Res* 2007; 20:32–6.
43. Guerrero-Romero F, Rodriguez-Moran M. Hypomagnesemia, oxidative stress, inflammation, and metabolic syndrome. *Diabetes Metab Res Rev* 2006; 22:471–6.
44. Rodriguez-Moran M, Guerrero-Romero F. Elevated concentrations of TNF-alpha are related to low serum magnesium levels in obese subjects. *Magnes Res* 2004; 17:189–96.
45. Mazur A, Maier JA, Rock E, Gueux E, Nowacki W, Rayssiguier Y. Magnesium and the inflammatory response: Potential physiopathological implications. *Arch Biochem Biophys* 2007; 458:48–56.
46. Weglicki WB, Mak IT, Kramer JH, Dickens BF, Cassidy MM, Stafford RE, et al. Role of free radicals and substance P in magnesium deficiency. *Cardiovasc Res* 1996; 31:677–82.
47. Hans CP, Chaudhary DP, Bansal DD. Effect of magnesium supplementation on oxidative stress in alloxanic diabetic rats. *Magnes Res* 2003; 16:13–9.
48. Yang Y, Wu Z, Chen Y, Qiao J, Gao M, Yuan J, et al. Magnesium deficiency enhances hydrogen peroxide production and oxidative damage in chick embryo hepatocyte in vitro. *Biometals* 2006; 19:71–81.
49. Afanas'ev IB, Suslova TB, Cheremisina ZP, Abramova NE, Korkina LG. Study of antioxidant properties of metal aspartates. *Analyst* 1995; 120:859–62.
50. Galland L. Magnesium and immune function: An overview. *Magnesium* 1988; 7:290–9.
51. Tam M, Gomez S, Gonzalez-Gross M, Marcos M. Possible roles of magne-sium on the immune system. *Eur J Clin Nutr* 2003; 57:1193–7.
52. Barbagallo M, Dominguez LJ, Galioto A, Ferlisi A, Cani C, Malfa L, et al. Role of magnesium in insulin action, diabetes and cardio-metabolic syn-drome X. *Mol Aspects Med* 2003; 24:39–52.
53. Barbagallo M, Dominguez LJ. Magnesium metabolism in hypertension and type 2 diabetes mellitus. *Am J Therapeutics* 2007; 14:375–85.
54. Touyz RM. Magnesium in clinical medicine. *Front Biosci* 2004; 9:1278–93.
55. Amighi J, Sabeti S, Schlager O, Mlekusch W, Exner M, Lalouschek W, et al. Low serum magnesium predicts neurological events in patients with advanced atherosclerosis. *Stroke* 2004; 35:22–7.
56. Shechter M, Merz CN, Rude RK, Paul Labrador MJ, Meisel SR, Shah PK, et al. Low intracellular magnesium levels promote platelet-dependent thrombo-sis in patients with coronary artery disease. *Am Heart J* 2000; 140:212–8.

57. Murck H. Magnesium and affective disorders. *Nutr Neurosci* 2002; 5:375–89.
58. Manuel Y, Keenoy B, Moorkens G, Vertommen J, Noe M, Neve J, De Leeuw I. Magnesium status and parameters of the oxidant-antioxidant balance in patients with chronic fatigue: Effects of supplementation with magnesium. *J Am Coll Nutr* 2000; 19:374–82.
59. Dominguez LJ, Barbagallo M, Di Lorenzo G, et al. Bronchial reactivity and intracellular magnesium: A possible mechanism for the bronchodilating effects of magnesium in asthma. *Clin Sci* 1998; 95:137–42.
60. He K, Liu K, Daviglus ML, Morris SJ, Loria CM, Van Horn L, et al. Magnesium intake and incidence of metabolic syndrome among young adults. *Circulation* 2006; 113:1675–82.
61. Resnick LM, Gupta RK, Bhargava KK, Gruenspan H, Alderman MH, Laragh JH. Cellular ions in hypertension, diabetes, and obesity: A nuclear magnetic resonance spectroscopic study. *Hypertension* 1991; 17:951–7.
62. Barbagallo M, Di Bella G, Brucato V, D'Angelo D, Damiani P, Monteverde A, Belvedere M, Dominguez LJ. Serum ionized magnesium in diabetic older persons. *Metabolism* 2014; 63:502–9.
63. Kao WH, Folsom AR, Nieto FJ, Mo JP, Watson RL, Brancati FL. Serum and dietary magnesium and the risk for type 2 diabetes mellitus: The Atherosclerosis Risk in Communities Study. *Arch Intern Med* 1999; 159:2151–9.
64. Matsunobu S, Terashima Y, Senshu T, Sano H, Itoh H. Insulin secretion and glucose uptake in hypomagnesemic sheep fed a low magnesium, high potassium diet. *J Nutr Biochem* 1990; 1:167–71.
65. Balon TW, Gu JL, Tokuyama Y, Jasman AP, Nadler JL. Magnesium supplementation reduces development of diabetes in a rat model of spontaneous NIDDM. *Am J Physiol* 1995; 269:E745–52.
66. Fung TT, Manson JE, Solomon CG, Liu S, Willett WC, Hu FB. The association between magnesium intake and fasting insulin concentration in healthy middle-aged women. *J Am Coll Nutr* 2003; 22:533–8.
67. Chaudhary DP, Boparai RK, Sharma R, Bansal DD. Studies on the development of an insulin resistant rat model by chronic feeding of low magnesium high sucrose diet. *Magnes Res* 2004; 17:293–300.
68. Barbagallo M, Dominguez LJ, Tagliamonte MR, Resnick LM, Paolisso G. Effects of vitamin E and glutathione on glucose metabolism: Role of magnesium. *Hypertension* 1999; 34:1002–6.
69. Paolisso G, D'Amore A, Balbi V, Volpe C, Galzerano D, Giugliano D, et al. Plasma vitamin C affects glucose homeostasis in healthy subjects and in non-insulin-dependent diabetics. *Am J Physiol* 1994; 266:E261–8.
70. Barbagallo M, Dominguez LJ, Tagliamonte MR, Resnick LM, Paolisso G. Effects of glutathione on red blood cell intracellular magnesium: Relation to glucose metabolism. *Hypertension* 1999; 34:76–82.
71. Lauretani F, Russo CR, Bandinelli S, Bartali B, Cavazzini C, Di Iorio A, et al. Age-associated changes in skeletal muscles and their effect on mobility: An operational diagnosis of sarcopenia. *J Appl Physiol* 2003; 95:1851–60.
72. Rock E, Astier C, Lab C, Vignon X, Gueux E, Motta C, et al. Dietary magnesium deficiency in rats enhances free radical production in skeletal muscle. *J Nutr* 1995; 125:1205–10.
73. Brilla LR, Haley TF. Effect of magnesium supplementation on strength training in humans. *J Am Coll Nutr* 1992; 11:326–9.

74. Brilla LR, Gunther KB. Effect of Mg supplementation on exercise time to exhaustion. *Med Exerc Nutr Health* 1995; 4:230.
75. Ter Borg S, de Groot L, Mijnarends D, de Vries J, Verlaan S, Meijboomb S, et al. Differences in nutrient intake and biochemical nutrient status between sarcopenic and nonsarcopenic older adults: Results from the Maastricht Sarcopenia Study. *JAMDA* 2016; 17:393–401.
76. Dominguez LJ, Barbagallo M, Lauretani F, Bandinelli S, Bos A, Corsi AM, et al. Magnesium and muscle performance in older persons: The InCHIANTI study. *Am J Clin Nutr* 2006; 84:419–26.
77. Veronese N, Berton L, Carraro S, Bolzetta F, De Rui M, Perissinotto E, et al, Effect of oral magnesium supplementation on physical performance in healthy elderly women involved in a weekly exercise program: A randomized controlled trial. *Am J Clin Nutr* 2014; 100:974–81.
78. Hartwig A. Role of magnesium in genomic stability. *Mutat Res* 2001; 475:113–21.
79. Rubin H. Central role for magnesium in coordinate control of metabolism and growth in animal cell. *Proc Natl Acad Sci USA* 1975; 72:3551–5.
80. McKeehan WL, Ham RG. Calcium and magnesium ions and the regulation of multiplication in normal and transformed cells. *Nature* 1978; 275:756–8.
81. Chien MM, Zahradka KE, Newell MK, Freed JH. Fas-induced B cell apoptosis requires an increase in free cytosolic magnesium as an early event. *J Biol Chem* 1999; 274:7059–66.
82. Dickens BF, Weglicki WB, Li YS, Mak IT. Magnesium deficiency in vitro enhances free radical-induced intracellular oxidation and cytotoxicity in endothelial cells. *FEBS Lett* 1992; 311:187–91.
83. Sgambato A, Wolf FI, Faraglia B, Cittadini A. Magnesium depletion causes growth inhibition, reduced expression of cyclin D1, and increased expression of P27Kip1 in normal but not in transformed mammary epithelial cells. *J Cell Physiol* 1999; 180:245–54.
84. Altura BM, Kostellow AB, Zhang A, Li W, Morrill GA, Gupta RK, Altura BT. Expression of the nuclear factor-kappa B and proto-oncogenes c-fos and c-jun are induced by low extracellular Mg2 in aortic and cerebral vascular smooth muscle cells: Possible links to hypertension, atherogenesis, and stroke. *Am J Hypertens* 2003; 16:701–7.
85. Killilea DA, Ames BM. Magnesium deficiency accelerates cellular senescence in cultured human fibroblasts. *PNAS-USA* 2008; 105:5768–73.

chapter four

Migraine and magnesium

Rebecca Michael and Jennifer S. Kriegler

Contents

Introduction

Migraine is a prevalent public health concern affecting 38 million men, women, and children in the United States and 1 billion individuals worldwide.[1] It is one of the leading causes of disability and has been associated with a significant impairment in quality of life.[2] The financial burden of migraine is also substantial, as it has been estimated to exceed $4 billion annually in health-care services and surpasses $14.5 billion every year for employers, secondary to reduced performance, decreased productivity, and absenteeism.[3]

The lack of a universally effective therapy and an incomplete understanding of migraine pathophysiology makes treatment challenging. Patients who are frustrated with conventional pharmacologic agents due to cost or lack of efficacy often turn to vitamins, minerals, and complementary and alternative medicine (CAM).[4]

There have been multiple mechanisms proposed in which magnesium is associated with migraine attacks. In several studies, magnesium deficiency has been associated with increased attacks.[5] However, magnesium supplementation in both the acute and preventive treatments of migraine has yielded mixed results. This chapter will further explore this interesting yet complex relationship between magnesium and migraine.

Migraine: The clinical phenotype

Migraine is an episodic disorder, the key feature of which is a moderate-to-severe headache generally associated with nausea and/or light and sound sensitivity. It also tends to be familial; the importance of inheritance in migraine has long been recognized. Migraine is further divided into migraine with aura and migraine without aura (Table 4.1). The frequency of the attacks also separates migraine into episodic and chronic forms. Chronic migraine (CM) is defined as migraine that occurs on 15 days/month or more for a minimum of 3 months. CM is the most disabling for patients and the most challenging for practitioners to manage.

Neurophysiological mechanism of migraine

The cause and mechanisms of migraine remain under constant investigation. Several theories have been proposed, including cortical spreading depression, trigeminovascular system involvement, central sensitization, and the role of serotonin and calcitonin gene-related peptide.

Table 4.1 ICHD-3 criteria

Migraine without Aura

At least five attacks fulfilling criteria 2 through 4
Headache lasting 4–72 hours (untreated or unsuccessfully treated)
Headache has at least two of the following characteristics:
- Unilateral location
- Pulsating quality
- Moderate or severe pain intensity
- Aggravation by causing avoidance of routine physical activity
During headache at least one of the following:
- Nausea, vomiting, or both
- Photophobia and phonophobia
Not better accounted for by another ICHD-3b diagnosis

Migraine with Aura

At least two attacks fulfilling criterion 2 and 3
One or more of the following fully reversible aura symptoms:
- Visual, sensory, speech and/or language, motor, brainstem, retinal
At least two of the following characteristics:
- Eat least one aura symptom spreads gradually over >5 minutes, and/or two or more symptoms occur in succession
- Each individual aura symptom lasts 5–60 minutes
- At least one aura symptom is unilateral
- The aura is accompanied, or following within 60 minutes, by headache
Not better accounted for by another ICHD-3b diagnosis, and transient ischemic attack has been excluded

The once-popular vascular theory of migraine, which suggested that migraine headache was caused by vasodilation, while the aura of migraine resulted from vasoconstriction, is no longer considered valid.[6] The dilation of blood vessels can occur; however, it is now felt to be a secondary phenomenon resulting from instability in the central neurovascular control mechanism.[6]

One theory that has been widely accepted and is relevant to magnesium's involvement in migraine is the cortical spreading depression theory of Leao.[7] Cortical spreading depression is a self-propagating wave of neuronal and glial depolarization that spreads across the cerebral cortex. It is thought that this phenomenon is the cause of the aura of migraine. The process of cortical spreading depression subsequently activates the trigeminal nerve afferents, which then causes inflammatory changes in the pain-sensitive meninges that produce the migraine headache through central and peripheral reflex mechanisms.[8]

It has also been suggested that migraine without aura may be caused by the occurrence of cortical spreading depression in regions of the brain (e.g., the cerebellum) in which depolarization is not consciously recognized.[9]

Biochemical role of magnesium in migraine

A large body of evidence exists on the importance of magnesium as an essential cation in biochemical and physiological processes in the human body. At least 325 enzymes are magnesium dependent, with many of these being brain enzymes.[10]

In the brain, magnesium binds to and inhibits N-methyl-D-aspartate (NMDA) glutamate receptors. NMDA excitatory receptors control the flux of cations across the neuronal membrane. Low magnesium can result in the opening of calcium channels, increasing intracellular calcium and extracellular potassium, subsequently resulting in glutamate release. It has been shown that the activation of cortical postsynaptic NMDA receptors helps propagate cortical spreading depression and aura. Therefore, low brain magnesium may be specifically associated with aura, suggesting magnesium is more likely to be effective in those with migraine with aura.[6]

There is also a proposed mechanism of the role of magnesium in the release of substance P,[11] stimulated cerebral artery spasm,[12] and an imbalance between mitochondrial energy production and demand.[13] Magnesium has also been shown to inhibit nociceptive trigeminal neurotransmission after microiontophoretic application in the trigeminocervical complex.[14]

Magnesium acute trials

A 2014 meta-analysis of five randomized controlled trials that evaluated intravenous magnesium for the acute treatment of migraine was unable to demonstrate a substantial effect on acute migraine attacks (30 minutes after treatment).[15] The meta-analysis excluded some frequently cited studies for methodological reasons and included only studies published in English, which could limit its external validity. A more recent meta-analysis of 13 trials demonstrated that intravenous magnesium yielded beneficial effects, alleviating acute migraine 15–45 minutes after the initial infusion. This analysis also demonstrated the intermediate (120 minutes) and long-term (24 hours) effects of intravenous magnesium on acute migraine.[2]

One independent study demonstrated pain relief in 88% of subjects within 15 minutes of infusion of 1 g of intravenous (IV) MgSO4. In this study, the patients with episodic migraine (compared with chronic migraine) and those with low ionized magnesium levels (0.54 mmol/L or lower) were more likely to respond. Eighty-nine percent of responders with 24-hour sustained pain-free response had low ionized magnesium; only 37.5% of non-responders had low ionized levels.[16]

Two additional studies have also demonstrated that patients with migraine with aura are more likely to respond to IV magnesium compared with those with migraine without aura.[15,17]

Magnesium prevention trials

Currently, the results of magnesium trials for the prevention of migraine are varied. Facchinetti and colleagues[18] studied 360 mg of elemental magnesium (as liquid magnesium pyrrolidone carboxylic acid) for the last two weeks of consecutive menstrual cycles and reported positive results compared with placebo for migraine intensity and duration. Peikert and colleagues[19] compared 600 mg of elemental magnesium (as trimagnesium dicitrate) with placebo daily for 12 weeks and found magnesium decreased attack frequency and the duration of attacks. Koseoglu and colleagues[20] studied 600 mg of elemental magnesium (as magnesium citrate) versus placebo in adult patients with migraine without aura and found positive results, with attack frequency decreasing from a median of three per month to two per month. Pfaffenrath and colleagues[21] compared placebo with 243 mg of elemental magnesium two times a day (as magnesium-L-aspartate-hydrochloride trihydrate). At interim analysis there was no difference between groups; therefore, the study was discontinued. Wang and colleagues[22] studied children ages 3–17 with migraine using 9 mg/kg of magnesium oxide. Only 73% completed the study, mostly because of the side effect of diarrhea. There was no significant difference in headache frequency from weeks 5–12.

A 2015 review of oral magnesium supplementation in migraine prevention showed that regardless of the various magnesium measurement techniques used, low magnesium levels and migraine largely remain associated.[3]

However, due to limited evidence, the authors suggested increasing dietary magnesium as a form of supplementation. The Canadian Headache Society guidelines for migraine prevention recommend 600 mg of elemental magnesium daily (as magnesium citrate), but the authors of this review suggested that it may be advantageous to consider dietary strategies to increase magnesium intake in individuals willing to make lifestyle changes, as these lifestyle modifications may also address other potential accompanying risk factors for migraine (e.g., obesity).[4]

Conclusion

Magnesium plays a role in migraine development at a biochemical level. There is a strong body of evidence demonstrating a relationship between magnesium status and migraine,[3] but the role of intravenous and oral magnesium supplementation in migraine treatment has yet to be fully elucidated. Additional randomized control trials evaluating this relationship are warranted.

Currently, the American Academy of Neurology/American Headache Society 2012 guidelines rated IV magnesium level B for acute migraine treatment,[22] while a 2014 meta-analysis suggests level U.[14] In addition, no standard dose has been established; however, either 1 g or 2 g in the form of MgSo4 is used most commonly.[23]

For the prevention of migraine the evidence is level B, with some positive studies for daily magnesium benefit in patients with aura and menstrual migraine. If magnesium supplementation is used, the recommended preventive dose is 400–600 mg per day for at least 3–4 months.[13] The most common adverse events seen with daily magnesium supplementation are flushing, diarrhea, and soft stools.

Bibliography

1. "Home: Migraine Research Foundation." Migraine Research Foundation. http://migraineresearchfoundation.org (accessed August 1, 2016).
2. Chiu, H.-Y., T.-H. Yeh, Y.-C. Huang, and P.-Y. Chen. "Effects of intravenous and oral magnesium on reducing migraine: a meta-analysis of randomized controlled trials." *Pain Physician*.2015; 19:97–112.
3. Teigen, L., and C. J. Boes. "An evidence-based review of oral magnesium supplementation in the preventative treatment of migraine." *Cephalgia*. 2015; 35:912–22.
4. Rajapakse, T., and T. Pringsheim. "Nutraceuticals in migraine: A summary of existing guidelines for use." *Headache: The Journal of Head and Face Pain*. 2016; 56(4):808–16.
5. Assarzadegan, F., S. Asgarzadeh, H. R. Hatamabadi, A. Shahrami, A. Tabatabaey, and M. Asgarzadeh. "Serum concentration of magnesium as an independent risk factor in migraine attacks." *International Clinical Psychopharmacology*. 2016; 31(5):287–92.

6. Charles, A. "Advances in the basic and clinical science of migraine." *Annals of Neurology.* 2009; 65(5):491–98.
7. Welch, K., G. D'Andrea, N. Tepley, G. Barkley, and N. M. Ramadan. "The concept of migraine as a state of central neuronal hyperexcitability." In *Neurologic Clinics: Headache,* 4th ed., Vol. 8, pp. 817–26. Philadelphia, PA: W.B. Saunders, 1990.
8. Bolay, H., U. Reuter, A. K. Dunn, et al. "Intrinsic brain activity triggers trigeminal meningeal afferents in a migraine model." *Nature Medicine.* 2002; 8:136.
9. Takano, T., and M. Nedergaard. "Deciphering migraine." *The Journal of Clinical Investigation.* 2009; 119:16.
10. Taylor, Frederick R. "Nutraceuticals and headache: The biological basis." *Headache: The Journal of Head and Face Pain.* 2011; 51(3): 484–501.
11. Weglicki, W. B., and T. M. Phillips. "Pathobiology of magnesium deficiency: A cytokine/neurogenic inflammation hypothesis." *The American Journal of Physiology.* 1992; 263:R734–37.
12. Schurks, M., J. E. Buring, and T. Kurth. "Migraine, migraine features, and cardiovascular disease." *Headache.* 2010; 50:1031–40.
13. Uncini, A., R. Lodi, A. Di Muzio, G. Silvestri, S. Servidei, A. Lugaresi, S. Iotti, P. Zaniol, and B. Barbiroli. "Abnormal brain and muscle energy metabolism shown by 31P-MRS in familial hemiplegic migraine." *Journal of the Neurological Sciences.* 1995; 129:214–22.
14. Tepper, Stewart J. "Nutraceutical and other modalities for the treatment of headache." *CONTINUUM: Lifelong Learning in Neurology.* 2015; 21:1018–31.
15. Choi, H., and N. Parmar. "The use of intravenous magnesium sulphate for acute migraine: Meta-analysis of randomized controlled trials." *European Journal of Emergency Medicine.* 2014; 21:2–9.
16. Mauksop, A., and J. Varughese. "Why all migraine patients should be treated with magnesium." *Journal of Neural Transmission (Vienna).* 2012; 119:575–79.
17. Bigal, M. E., C. A. Bordini, S. J. Tepper, J. G. Speciali. "Intravenous magnesium sulfate in the acute treatment of migraine without aura and migraine with aura: A randomized double-blind, placebo-controlled study." *Cephalgia.* 2002; 22(5):345-53.
18. Facchinetti, F., G. Sances, P. Borella, A. R. Genazzani, and G. Nappi. "Magnesium prophylaxis of menstrual migraine: Effects on intracellular magnesium." *Headache: The Journal of Head and Face Pain.* 1991; 31(5):298–301.
19. Peikert, A., C. Wilimzig, and R. Kohne-Volland. "Prophylaxis of migraine with oral magnesium: Results from a prospective, multi-center, placebo-controlled and double-blind randomized study." *Cephalalgia.* 1996; 16(4):257–63.
20. Koseoglu, E., A. Talaslioglu, A. S. Gonol, and M. Kula. "The effects of magnesium prophylaxis in migraine without aura." *Magnesium Research.* 2008; 21:101–8.
21. Pfaffenrath, V., P. Wessely, C. Meyer, H. R. Isler, S. Evers, K. H. Grotemeyer, Z. Taneri, D. Soyka, H. Gobel, and M. Fischer. "Magnesium in the prophylaxis of migraine: A double-blind, placebo-controlled study." *Cephalalgia.* 1996; 16(6):436–40.
22. Wang, F., S. K. Van Den Eeden, L. M. Ackerson, S. E. Salk, R. H. Reince, and R. J. Elin. "Oral magnesium oxide prophylaxis of frequent migrainous headache in children: A randomized, double-blind, placebo-controlled trial." *Headache: The Journal of Head and Face Pain.* 2003; 43(6):601–10.

23. Mauskop, A., S. Holland, S. D. Silberstein, F. Freitag, D. W. Dodick, and C. Argoff. "Evidence-based guideline update: NSAIDs and other complementary treatments for episodic migraine prevention in adults: Report of the Quality Standards Subcommittee of the American Academy of Neurology and the American Headache Society." *Neurology.* 2013; 80(9):868–69.

24. Soma Sahai-Srivastava, M. D., and M. S. Tanya Jain Gupta. "Magnesium sulfate in the treatment of acute migraine headaches." *Practical Pain Management.* http://www.practicalpainmanagement.com/treatments/pharmacological/non-opioids/magnesium-sulfate-helpful-treatment-acute-migraines (accessed August 1, 2016).

25. Storer, R. J., and P. J. Goadsby. "N-methyl-D-aspartate receptor channel complex blockers including memantine and magnesium inhibit nociceptive traffic in the trigeminocervical complex of the rat." *Cephalgia.* 2009; 29 (suppl 1):135.

26. Hoffmann, J., J. W. Park, R. J. Storer, and P. J. Goadsby. "Magnesium and memantine do not inhibit nociceptive neuronal activity in the trigeminocervical complex of the rat." *The Journal of Headache and Pain.* 2013; 14 (suppl 1):P71.

27. Mauskop, A., B. T. Altura, R. Q. Cracco, and B. M. Altura. "Intravenous magnesium sulfate rapidly alleviates headaches of various types." *Headache.* 1996; 36(3):154–60.

28. Rybicka, M., I. Baranowska-Bosiacka, B. Zyluk, P. Nowacki, and D. Chlubek. "The role of magnesium in migraine pathogenesis: Potential use of magnesium compounds in prevention and treatment of migraine headaches." *Journal of Elementology.* 2012; 17:345–56.

29. Welch, K. M., and N. M. Ramadan. "Mitochondria, magnesium and migraine." *Journal of the Neurological Sciences.* 1995; 134:9–14.

chapter five

Magnesium and dyslipidemia

Fernando Guerrero-Romero and Martha Rodríguez-Morán

Contents

Introduction

According to the National Health and Nutrition Examination Survey (NHANES) 1999–2010, the prevalence of dyslipidemia was 49.7%, 44.2%, and 28.6% among U.S. adults with obesity, overweight, and normal weight, respectively.[1] This pattern of dyslipidemia is consistent worldwide. The Indian Council of Medical Research–India Diabetes study conducted the prevalence of hypercholesterolemia, hypertriglyceridemia, low HDL-c, and high LDL-c levels in a representative population of three states of India and one Union Territory covering a population of 213 million people. They found that 13.9%, 29.5%, 72.3%, and 11.8%, respectively, had hypercholesterolemia, hypertriglyceridemia, low HDL-c, and high LDL-c levels, with 79% of the subjects studied exhibiting abnormalities in one of the lipid parameters.[2] The prevalence of dyslipidemia in adults of Uygur, Kazak, and Han ethnicity in Xinjiang, China was 52.6%, 35.4%, and 33.2%, respectively. In addition, differences in the standardized prevalence rates of high triglycerides (9.3%, 9.3%, and 17.3%), high total cholesterol (5.2%, 6.9%, and 6%), low HDL-c (33.6%, 20.8%, and 11.1%), and high LDL-c (2.4%, 2.9%, and 2%), were also seen.[3] Among Turkish adults, the prevalence of total cholesterol, low HDL-c, high LDL-c, and high triglycerides levels is 43%, 41.5%, 36.2%, and 35.7%, respectively.[4] In Spain, the results of the Di@bet.es study, a national population-based survey, show a prevalence of dyslipidemia of 56.8% among adults,[5] whereas in the DYSIS-Middle East study, a study from the United Arab Emirates (UAE), Saudi Arabia, Lebanon, and Jordan, the prevalence of low HDL-c and elevated triglycerides were 55.5% and 48.5%, respectively.[6] Finally, Frank et al.[7] showed that in Northern California, minority groups, excluding African Americans, were more likely to have high triglyceride/low HDL-c. Irrespective of racial/ethnic differences, dyslipidemia is a cardiovascular risk factor with high prevalence across different cohorts. Nonetheless, the findings of these studies emphasize the role of genes in the development of dyslipidemia and the need to determine how race and ethnicity affect differences in cardiovascular disease rates.[7]

Although dyslipidemia is highly prevalent among obese individuals, some individuals show a phenotypic variant of metabolically obese but normal weight (MONW). This is characterized by normal-weight individuals eliciting obesity-related phenotypic characteristics, such as insulin resistance, hyperglycemia, hypertriglyceridemia, and/or high blood pressure.[8,9] The prevalence of MONW is high, and NHANES 1999–2004 and NHANES 1999–2010 showed that the prevalence of MONW was 23.5% and 28.6%, respectively.[10,11] In Mexican individuals from northern Mexico, the prevalence of MONW is 48.5%,[12] and in the Asian population varies from 12.7% to 13.3%.[13,14] These findings support the hypothesis that health behaviors, in addition to the role of ethnicity, are involved in the development of dyslipidemia in normal-weight individuals. So, irrespective of body weight, the prevalence of dyslipidemia is high.

In addition to urgent lifestyle interventions, new strategies to prevent this important cardiovascular risk factor are necessary. Among these strategies is the need for a better understanding of the role of magnesium in the pathogenesis of dyslipidemia. A recent cross-sectional study reported that hypomagnesemia was associated with the presence of metabolic abnormalities (adjusted odds ratio [OR] 6.4; 95% CI 2.3–20.4), supporting the possible role of magnesium in the pathways leading to the development of dyslipidemia.

In this chapter, we review evidence showing the link between hypomagnesemia and dyslipidemia.

Role of magnesium in the pathophysiology of dyslipidemia

Magnesium, the most abundant intracellular divalent cation[15,16] and the second-most abundant intracellular cation,[17] is an essential co-factor in the enzymatic process of high-energy phosphate production,[18,19] the synthesis of nucleic acids and proteins, cytoskeletal function, cell cycle progression, the maintenance of membrane integrity and stability, ion homeostasis,[20] and glucose-related metabolic pathways.[21,22] The anti-atherogenic effects of magnesium appear to involve the modification of several enzymes intricately linked with lipid metabolism, inhibiting the activity of lecithin cholesterol acyl transferase (LCAT) and HMG-CoA reductase, and stimulating the activity of lipoprotein lipase.[23] Magnesium is necessary for activity of LCAT, which lowers LDL-C and triglyceride levels and raises HDL-C levels; it has been reported that rodents fed magnesium-deficient diets have higher serum triglyceride levels and reduced HDL-c secondary to the reduction of serum activity of LCAT.[24] LCAT is also involved in reverse cholesterol uptake, facilitating cholesterol uptake from tissues into HDL-c.[25] Experimental studies conducted in rats show that severe magnesium deficiency produces marked changes in the fatty acid pattern of total plasma lipids.[26] Furthermore, the enzyme that deactivates HMG-CoA reductase requires magnesium; *in vitro* studies show that increasing the content of magnesium in bathing solution attenuates HMG-CoA reductase activity.[27]

In addition to the modulation of the aforementioned enzymes, experimental studies show that VLDL + LDL particles from magnesium-deficient rats were more susceptible to oxidative damage than lipoproteins from control rats, suggesting that the mechanism responsible for atherogenicity and tissue damage, characteristic of magnesium deficiency, could be mediated by an increased susceptibility of triglyceride-rich lipoproteins to peroxidation.[28] Uehara et al.[29] showed that magnesium-deficient rats exhibit increased levels of phosphati-dylcholine hydroperoxide, a primary product of lipid peroxidation in biological membranes, plasma, and several tissues. Finally, it has been shown that inadequate magnesium intake results in an increase of atherosclerotic plaque development in rabbits,[30] supporting the hypothesis that dietary magnesium intake and serum magnesium levels are inversely correlated with the development of atherosclerosis.

Hypomagnesemia could therefore promote the development of dyslipidemia by altering the catalytic activity of several enzymes involved in lipid metabolism and promoting the oxidation of serum lipids.[23] Taken together, all these studies indicate and support the hypothesis that magnesium, at optimal cellular concentration, has effects that parallel those of statins, and could be considered a physiological statin in the reduction of lipids.[31]

Evidence linking magnesium deficiency with dyslipidemia

Results from experimental studies show that a magnesium-rich diet could exert a cardioprotective effect by reducing the plasma's total cholesterol and triglycerides levels, and the ameliorating HDL-c/total cholesterol ratio in diabetic rats.[32] In addition, it has been shown that increased magnesium intake reduces lipid peroxidation and improves hyperlipidemia in fructose-fed rats.[33] In female rat models with dyslipidemia associated with the use of oral contraceptives, rats who received a high magnesium intake had higher plasma HDL-c levels, lower LDL-c levels, and lower atherogenic indices,[34] suggesting that dyslipidemia associated with oral contraceptive use may be prevented by supplementary dietary magnesium intake.

In addition, Shah et al.[35] found that short-term dietary magnesium deficiency in rats would result in the reduction of HDL-c, concomitant with elevations in total cholesterol, LDL + VLDL, and triglycerides levels. Consistently with the results of Shah et al.,[35] Spasov et al.[36] demonstrated that magnesium deficiency in rats resulted in higher triglyceride levels (by 35.2%), LDL-c (more than fourfold), total cholesterol (by 38.7%), and lower HDL-c (by 28.7%). In this study, Spasov et al.[36] showed that oral magnesium salts (magnesium L-aspartate and magnesium chloride) led to the normalization of the lipid profile with a return to pre-deficient levels. In the same way, the results by Takeda et al.[37] show that the increase of magnesium intake reduces plasma lipid parameters such as cholesterol and triglycerides in female Wistar rats. These results suggest that higher magnesium intake, by reducing lipid indices, might have a prophylactic potential effect against the onset of hyperlipidemia and cardiovascular disease.[37]

Clinical studies have revealed that magnesium deficiency correlates with cardiovascular risk factors including insulin resistance, dyslipidemia, and inflammatory reaction that leads to atherosclerosis in both diabetic and non-diabetic individuals.[38-40] Among diabetic individuals with hypomagnesemia, hypertriglyceridemia is pronounced, suggesting that low serum magnesium and high triglycerides levels could be a reliable biochemical marker of insulin status, without resorting to the use of criteria for insulin sensitivity.[39] Also, magnesium shows a positive correlation with HDL-c levels and is negatively correlated with total cholesterol and LDL-c in diabetic patients, supporting the hypothesis that hypomagnesemia is accompanied by atherogenic alterations in the lipid profiles of type 2 diabetic patients.[38] These findings support the notion that magnesium supplementation may be needed in individuals with type 2 diabetes. However, Nasri et al.[41] reported significant inverse correlations of serum magnesium with serum cholesterol and LDL-c but no significant correlations of serum magnesium with HDL-c and triglycerides. In a large adult study population of healthy individuals, serum magnesium was positively correlated with total cholesterol, HDL-c, LDL-c, and triglyceride levels, suggesting that serum magnesium and serum lipid levels may be different in healthy individuals compared with those with diabetes.[40]

Results from dietary interventional studies are controversial. Aslanabadi et al.,[42] who conducted a randomized controlled trial to evaluate the efficacy of a mineral water (rich in calcium, magnesium bicarbonate, and sulfate) versus spring water (with a composition similar to that of urban water) on the lipid profile of dyslipidemic adults showed that an intake of mineral water rich in magnesium bicarbonate for 1 month decreased cholesterol and LDL-c levels but not triglycerides or HDL-c levels. In another study, the consumption of spring water rich in magnesium showed no significant effects on serum lipids in postmenopausal women after 84 days of the intake of mineral water.[43] In addition, a 6-week study looking at the consumption of filtered and reverse-osmosed deep seawater (containing 395 mg/dL of elemental magnesium) versus magnesium-chloride-fortified water to decrease serum lipids in hypercholesterolemic subjects showed a progressive decrease in total serum cholesterol and LDL-c levels in the group that consumed deep sea water.[44] However, deep seawater also is rich in other minerals and trace elements such as sulfate, lithium, selenium, molybdenum, silicon, and zinc. Thus, magnesium content could not be a sole factor behind the hypocholesterolemic effect.[44]

Kishimoto et al.[45] determined the effects of magnesium supplementation on postprandial responses in serum lipid levels using bittern, a natural magnesium chloride solution from sea water. They enrolled 16 healthy males in a two-way, randomized crossover study; participants consumed 30 g of butter with or without 5 ml of bittern containing 500 mg of magnesium. Serum and T-chylomicron triglycerides levels were reduced and delayed by magnesium supplementation. The authors concluded that magnesium supplementation could inhibit fat absorption and improve postprandial hyperlipidemia in healthy subjects.

Other dietary interventional studies have been focused on the use of almonds. It is well known that almonds, peanuts, macadamia nuts, hazelnuts, pistachios, and pecans are low in saturated fatty acids, rich in unsaturated fatty acids, and contain fiber, phytosterols, plant protein, α-tocopherol, resveratrol, phenolic compounds, arginine, magnesium, copper, manganese, calcium, and potassium.[46–48] Although there is a remarkable consistency among epidemiological studies regarding the higher frequency of nut intake and reduced risk of heart disease,[49,50] controlled studies to demonstrate its beneficial effect on lipid profile are scarce.[47,51,52] A small 12-week randomized crossover clinical trial conducted in diabetic patients showed that almonds added to replace 20% of total daily calorie intake decreased total cholesterol, LDL-c, and the ratio of LDL-c/HDL-c 6.0%, 11.6%, and 9.7%, respectively.[51] In a small randomized crossover design study, in which the experimental diets included (1) Step I diet, (2) low-almond diet, and (3) high-almond diet (almonds contributing 0%, 10%, and 20% of total energy, respectively), the incorporation of approximately 68 g of almonds (20% of energy) markedly improved the serum lipid profile of healthy and mildly hypercholesterolemic adults. Total and LDL-c levels declined with progressively higher intakes of almonds, which suggests a dose–response relation.[53] Because almonds have many other micronutrients, it is uncertain if the magnesium alone had any role to play. Yet, the combination of these micronutrients (vitamins C and E with magnesium and zinc) have been evaluated in type 2 diabetic patients and was found to significantly increase HDL-c levels but had no effects on the serum levels of total cholesterol, LDL-c, and triglycerides.[54]

Rajaram et al.[52] enrolled 23 individuals in a single-blind, randomized, controlled crossover feeding study to evaluate the efficacy of pecans rich in monounsaturated fat as an alternative to modifying serum lipids and lipoproteins in men and women with normal to moderately high serum cholesterol levels. After 4 weeks of feeding a pecan-enriched diet, serum total cholesterol, LDL-c, and triglycerides decreased 6.7%, 10.4%, and 11.1%, respectively.

Prospective randomized double-blind control trials to evaluate the efficacy of magnesium supplementation on lipid profile are scarce.[55,56] Shechter et al.[56] conducted a randomized, prospective, double-blind cross-over study with 41 healthy volunteers to evaluate the impact of supplemental oral magnesium citrate versus magnesium oxide. They found that oral magnesium oxide rather than magnesium citrate reduced total cholesterol and LDL-c levels.

Recently, our group enrolled 47 MONW individuals with hypomagnesemia in a randomized double-blind placebo-controlled clinical trial.[56] Subjects in the experimental group received magnesium chloride (equivalent to 382 mg of magnesium) once daily for 4 months and were compared with a control placebo group. Subjects that received magnesium experienced a significant decrease in blood pressure, fasting glucose, HOMA-IR index, and triglyceride levels (-47.4% vs. 10.1%, $p < 0.0001$). Our results strongly suggest that oral magnesium supplementation may be useful in improving the metabolic profile of normal-weight individuals with dyslipidemia.[56]

Conclusions

Although results from experimental and epidemiological studies show a consistent inverse relationship between serum magnesium and total cholesterol, LDL-c, and triglyceride levels, and a direct relationship between serum magnesium with HDL-c levels, results from dietary interventional studies are controversial. Some studies show a beneficial effect, but others do not. Though few randomized double-blind clinical trials evaluating the effect of oral magnesium supplementation on the lipid profile have shown consistent results, there is not yet enough robust data in support of any recommendation in relation to dietary modification using magnesium supplementation. Nevertheless, the consumption of almonds, peanuts, macadamia nuts, hazelnuts, pistachios, and pecans by healthy individuals and diabetic patients should be encouraged. There is an urgent need for further research in this field.

References

1. Saydah S, Bullard KM, Cheng Y, Ali MK, Gregg EW, Geiss L, Imperatore G. Trends in cardiovascular disease risk factors by obesity level in adults in the United States, NHANES1999–2010. *Obesity (Silver Spring)* 2014;22:1888–95.
2. Joshi SR, Anjana RM, Deepa M, Pradeepa R, Bhansali A, Dhandania VK, Joshi PP, et al.; ICMR–INDIAB Collaborative Study Group. Prevalence of dyslipidemia in urban and rural India: The ICMR-INDIAB study. *PLoS One* 2014;9:e96808.
3. Guo SX, Ma RL, Guo H, Ding YS, Liu JM, Zhang M, Zhang JY, et al. Epidemiological analysis of dyslipidemia in adults of three ethnicities in Xinjiang, China. *Genet Mol Res* 2014;13:2385–93.
4. Bayram F, Kocer D, Gundogan K, Kaya A, Demir O, Coskun R, Sabuncu T, et al. Prevalence of dyslipidemia and associated risk factors in Turkish adults. *J Clin Lipidol* 2014;8:206–16.
5. Martinez-Hervas S, Carmena R, Ascaso JF, Real JT, Masana L, Catalá M, Vendrell J, et al. Prevalence of plasma lipid abnormalities and its association with glucose metabolism in Spain: The di@bet.es study. *Clin Investig Arterioscler* 2014;26(3):107–14.
6. Al Sifri SN, Almahmeed W, Azar S, Okkeh O, Bramlage P, Jünger C, Halawa I, Ambegaonkar B, Wajih S, Brudi P. Results of the Dyslipidemia International Study (DYSIS)-Middle East: Clinical perspective on the prevalence and characteristics of lipid abnormalities in the setting of chronic statin treatment. *PLoS One.* 2014;9:e84350.
7. Frank AT, Zhao B, Jose PO, Azar KM, Fortmann SP, Palaniappan LP. Racial/ethnic differences in dyslipidemia patterns. *Circulation* 2014;129:570–9.
8. Conus F, Rabasa-Lhoret R, Péronnet F. Characteristics of metabolically obese normal-weight (MONW) subjects. *Appl Physiol Nutr Metab* 2007;32:4–12.
9. St-Onge MP, Janssen I, Heymsfield SB. Metabolic syndrome in normal-weight Americans: New definition of the metabolically obese, normal-weight individual. *Diabetes Care* 2004;27:2222–8.
10. Wildman RP, Muntner P, Reynolds K, McGinn AP, Rajpathak S, Wylie-Rosett J, et al. The obese without cardiometabolic risk factor clustering and the normal weight with cardiometabolic risk factor clustering: Prevalence and correlates of 2 phenotypes among the US population (NHANES 1999–2004). *Arch Intern Med* 2008;168:1617–24.
11. Gregg EW, Cheng YJ, Cadwell BL, Imperatore G, Williams DE, Flegal KM, Narayan KM, Williamson DF. Secular trends in cardiovascular disease risk factors according to body mass index in US adults. *JAMA* 2005;293:1868–74.
12. Guerrero-Romero F, Rodriguez-Moran M. Serum magnesium in the metabolically-obese normal-weight and healthy-obese subjects. *Eur J Intern Med* 2013;24:639–43.
13. Geetha L, Deepa M, Anjana RM, Mohan V. Prevalence and clinical profile of metabolic obesity and phenotypic obesity in Asian Indians. *J Diabetes Sci Technol* 2011;5:439–46.
14. Lee K. Metabolically obese but normal weight (MONW) and metabolically healthy but obese (MHO) phenotypes in Koreans: Characteristics and health behaviors. *Asia Pac J Clin Nutr* 2009;18:280–84.
15. Lopez Martinez J, Sanchez Castilla M, Garcia de Lorenzo y Mateos A, Culebras Fernandez JM. Magnesium: Metabolism and requirements. *Nutr Hosp* 1997;12:4–14.

16. Grubbs RD, Maguire ME. Magnesium as a regulatory cation: Criteria and evaluation. *Magnesium* 1987;6:113–27.
17. Touyz RM. Magnesium in clinical medicine. *Front Bio Sci* 2004;9:1278–93.
18. Garfinkel D, Garfinkel L. Magnesium and regulation of carbohydrate metabolism at the molecular level. *Magnesium* 1988;7:249–61.
19. Paolisso G, Scheen A, D'Onofrio F, Lefèbvre P. Magnesium and glucose homeostasis. *Diabetologia* 1990;33:511–4.
20. Saris NE, Mervaala E, Karppanen H, Khawaja JA, Lewenstam A. Magnesium: An update on physiological, clinical and analytical aspects. *Clin Chim Acta* 2000;294:1–26.
21. Paolisso G, Barbagallo M. Hypertension, diabetes mellitus, and insulin resistance: The role of intracellular magnesium. *Am J Hypertens* 1997;10:346–55.
22. Laughlin MR, Thompson D. The regulatory role for magnesium in glycolytic flux of the human erythrocyte. *J Biol Chem* 1996;271:28977–83.
23. Belin RJ, He K. Magnesium physiology and pathogenic mechanisms that contribute to the development of the metabolic syndrome. *Magnes Res* 2007;20:107–29.
24. Touyz RM, Panz V, Milne FJ. Relations between magnesium, calcium, and plasma renin activity in black and white hypertensive patients. *Miner Electrolyte Metab* 1995;21:417–22.
25. Jonas A. Lecithin cholesterol acyltransferase. *Biochim Biophys Acta* 2000;1529:245–56.
26. Rayssiguier Y. Magnesium, lipids and vascular diseases: Experimental evidence in animal models. *Magnesium* 1986;5:182–90.
27. Field FJ, Henning B, Mathur SN. In vitro regulation of 3-hydroxy-3-methylglutarylcoenzyme A reductase and acylcoenzyme A: Cholesterol acyltransferase activities by phosphorylation-dephosphorylation in rabbit intestine. *Biochim Biophys Acta* 1984;802:9–16
28. Gueux E, Cubizolles C, Bussière L, Mazur A, Rayssiguier Y. Oxidative modification of triglyceride-rich lipoproteins in hypertriglyceridemic rats following magnesium deficiency. *Lipids* 1993;28:573–5.
29. Uehara M, Chiba H, Fujii A, Masuyama R, Suzuki K. Induction of phospholipid hydroperoxides in relation to change of tissue mineral distribution caused by magnesium-deficiency in rats. In: Rayssiguier Y, Mazur, Durlach J, eds. *Advances in Magnesium Research: Nutrition and Health*. Paris: John Libbey Eurotext, 2001: 291–6.
30. King JL, Miller RJ, Blue JP, Jr, O'Brien WD, Jr, Erdman JW, Jr. Inadequate dietary magnesium intake increases atherosclerotic plaque development in rabbits. *Nutr Res* 2009;29:343–9.
31. Rosanoff A, Seelig MS. Comparison of mechanism and functional effects of magnesium and statin pharmaceuticals. *J Am Coll Nutr* 2004;23:501S–5S.
32. Olatunji LA, Soladoye AO. Effect of increased magnesium intake on plasma cholesterol, triglyceride and oxidative stress in alloxan-diabetic rats. *Afr J Med Med Sci* 2007;36:155–61.
33. Olatunji LA, Soladoye AO. Increased magnesium intake prevents hyperlipidemia and insulin resistance and reduces lipid peroxidation in fructose-fed rats. *Pathophysiology* 2007;14:11–5.
34. Olatunji LA, Oyeyipo IP, Micheal OS, Soladoye AO. Effect of dietary magnesium on glucose tolerance and plasma lipid during oral contraceptive administration in female rats. *Afr J Med Med Sci* 2008;37:135–9.

35. Shah NC, Liu JP, Iqbal J, Hussain M, Jiang XC, Li Z, Li Y, et al. Mg deficiency results in modulation of serum lipids, glutathione, and NO synthase isozyme activation in cardiovascular tissues: Relevance to de novo synthesis of ceramide, serum Mg and atherogenesis. *Int J Clin Exp Med* 2011;4:103–18.
36. Spasov AA, Iezgitsa IN, Kharitonova MV, Kravchenko MS. Effect of some organic and inorganic magnesium salts on lipoprotein state in rats fed with magnesium-deficient diet. *Eksp Klin Farmakol* 2008;71:35–40.
37. Takeda R, Nakamura T. Effects of high magnesium intake on bone mineral status and lipid metabolism in rats. *J Nutr Sci Vitaminol (Tokyo)* 2008;54:66–75.
38. Rasheed H, Elahi S, Ajaz H. Serum magnesium and atherogenic lipid fractions in type II diabetic patients of Lahore, Pakistan. *Biol Trace Elem Res* 2012;148:165–9.
39. Srinivasan AR, Niranjan G, Kuzhandai Velu V, Parmar P, Anish A. Status of serum magnesium in type 2 diabetes mellitus with particular reference to serum triacylglycerol levels. *Diabetes Metab Syndr* 2012;6:1879.
40. Randell EW, Mathews M, Gadag V, Zhang H, Sun G. Relationship between serum magnesium values, lipids and anthropometric risk factors. *Atherosclerosis* 2008;196:413–9.
41. Nasri H, Baradaran HR. Lipids in association with serum magnesium in diabetes mellitus patients. *Bratisl Lek Listy* 2008;109:302–6.
42. Aslanabadi N, Habibi Asl B, Bakhshalizadeh B, Ghaderi F, Nemati M. Hypolipidemic activity of a natural mineral water rich in calcium, magnesium, and bicarbonate in hyperlipidemic adults. *Adv Pharm Bull* 2014;4:303–7.
43. Day RO, Liauw W, Tozer LM, McElduff P, Beckett RJ, Williams KM. A double-blind, placebo-controlled study of the short term effects of a spring water supplemented with magnesium bicarbonate on acid/base balance, bone metabolism and cardiovascular risk factors in postmenopausal women. *BMC Res Notes* 2010;3:180.
44. Fu ZY, Yang FL, Hsu HW, Lu YF. Drinking deep seawater decreases serum total and low-density lipoprotein-cholesterol in hypercholesterolemic subjects. *J Med Food* 2012;15:535–41.
45. Kishimoto Y, Tani M, Uto-Kondo H, Saita E, Iizuka M, Sone H, Yokota K, Kondo K. Effects of magnesium on postprandial serum lipid responses in healthy human subjects. *Br J Nutr* 2010;103:469–72.
46. Berryman CE, Preston AG, Karmally W, Deckelbaum RJ, Kris-Etherton PM. Effects of almond consumption on the reduction of LDL-cholesterol: A discussion of potential mechanisms and future research directions. *Nutr Rev* 2011;69:171–85.
47. Sabaté J, Wien M. Nuts, blood lipids and cardiovascular disease. *Asia Pac J Clin Nutr* 2010;19:131–6.
48. Kris-Etherton PM, Hu FB, Ros E, Sabaté J. The role of tree nuts and peanuts in the prevention of coronary heart disease: Multiple potential mechanisms. *J Nutr* 2008;138:1746S–51S.
49. Fraser GE, Shavlik DJ. Risk factors for all-cause and coronary heart disease mortality in the oldest-old: The Adventist Health Study. *Arch Intern Med* 1997;157:2249–58.
50. Hu FB, Stampfer MJ, Manson JE, Rimm EB, Colditz GA, Rosner BA, Speizer FE, Hennekens CH, Willett WC. Frequent nut consumption and risk of coronary heart disease in women: Prospective cohort study. *BMJ* 1998;317:1341–5.

51. Li SC, Liu YH, Liu JF, Chang WH, Chen CM, Chen CY. Almond consumption improved glycemic control and lipid profiles in patients with type 2 diabetes mellitus. *Metabolism* 2011;60:474–9.
52. Rajaram S, Burke K, Connell B, Myint T, Sabaté J. A monounsaturated fatty acid-rich pecan-enriched diet favorably alters the serum lipid profile of healthy men and women. *J Nutr* 2001;131:2275–9.
53. Sabaté J, Haddad E, Tanzman JS, Jambazian P, Rajaram S. Serum lipid response to the graduated enrichment of a Step I diet with almonds: A randomized feeding trial. *Am J Clin Nutr* 2003;77:1379–84.
54. Farvid MS, Siassi F, Jalali M, Hosseini M, Saadat N. The impact of vitamin and/or mineral supplementation on lipid profiles in type 2 diabetes. *Diabetes Res Clin Pract* 2004;65:21–8.
55. Shechter M, Saad T, Shechter A, Koren-Morag N, Silver BB, Matetzky S. Comparison of magnesium status using X-ray dispersion analysis following magnesium oxide and magnesium citrate treatment of healthy subjects. *Magnes Res* 2012;25:28–39.
56. Guerrero-Romero F, Rodríguez-Moran M. Oral magnesium supplementation improves the metabolic profile of metabolically-obese, normal-weight individuals: A randomized double-blind placebo-controlled trial. *Arch Med Res* 2014;45:388–93.

chapter six

Magnesium and the metabolic syndrome

Fernando Guerrero-Romero and Martha Rodríguez-Morán

Contents

Introduction

The metabolic syndrome is a cluster of metabolic risk factors that include obesity, hyperglycemia, dyslipidemia (characterized by high triglyceride and low high-density lipoprotein [HDL] cholesterol levels), and elevated blood pressure.[1] This syndrome is of particular importance given its large prevalence in the general population worldwide and because it is a predisposing condition that increases the risk of cardiovascular disease and diabetes mellitus.[2,3] Individuals with metabolic syndrome are at twice the risk for cardiovascular disease compared with those without. It also raises the risk for type 2 diabetes by about fivefold.[4]

In order to implement appropriate preventive strategies for cardiovascular disease, it is important to recognize the presence of the risk factors and their relevance to the development of metabolic syndrome. However, the main problem with studying metabolic syndrome in the general population is that academic groups have postulated their own definitions, which leads to differences in the estimation of its prevalence.[5-7] According to some experts, the main criticism of metabolic syndrome's definition is that aggregating metabolic risk factors into a syndrome would add little to the patient's clinical management. The counterargument emphasizes that the clustering of risk factors changes the clinical focus of therapies to targeting underlying causes.[8] Among the most accepted and used definitions of the metabolic syndrome are those from the Third Report of the National Cholesterol Education Program (NCEP) Expert Panel on Detection, Evaluation, and Treatment of High Blood Cholesterol in Adults (Adult Treatment Panel III; ATPIII) [1] and the International Diabetes Federation (IDF).[9,10] According to the ATPIII criteria, any three or more of the following five components are required for the diagnosis of metabolic syndrome: obesity (waist circumference equal to or greater than 102 cm in men and 88 cm in women), hypertriglyceridemia (triglycerides levels equal to or greater than 150 mg/dL), low HDL (equal or lower than 40 mg/dL in men and equal to or lower than 50 mg/dL in women), hyperglycemia (fasting glucose equal to or greater than 110 mg/dL), and high blood pressure (systolic and diastolic blood pressures equal to or greater than 130 and 85 mmHg, respectively).[1] IDF criteria[9] requires the presence of central obesity (equal to or greater than 94 cm for European men and equal to or greater than 80 cm for European women, with ethnicity-specific values for other groups in Table 6.1, plus any two of the following risk factors: hypertriglyceridemia (triglycerides levels equal to or greater than 150 mg/dL), low HDL (equal to or lower than 40 mg/dL in men and equal to or lower than 50 mg/dL in women, and/or specific treatment for this lipid abnormality in both males and females), hyperglycemia (fasting glucose equal to or greater than 100 mg/dL, or previously diagnosed type 2 diabetes), and high blood pressure (systolic and diastolic blood pressures equal to or greater than 130 and 85 mmHg, respectively). Although the obesity epidemic is largely responsible for the high prevalence of the metabolic syndrome, the main difference between the ATPIII and IDF definitions is that the IDF's criteria take into account the presence of obesity and then the other cardiovascular risk factors. Based on the IDF criteria,

Table 6.1 Ethnic cut-off values for diagnosis of obesity, based in waist circumference, according to criteria by the IDF

Ethnic group	Male	Female
Europids	≥94 cm	≥80 cm
United States	≥102 cm	≥88 cm
South Asians	≥90 cm	≥80 cm
Chinese	≥90 cm	≥80 cm
Japanese	≥90 cm	≥80 cm
South and Central Americans	≥90 cm	≥80 cm
Sub-Saharan Africans	≥94 cm	≥80 cm
Eastern Mediterraneans	≥94 cm	≥80 cm
Middle East (Arab)	≥94 cm	≥80 cm

it is not possible to recognize the presence of metabolic syndrome among metabolically obese, normal-weight individuals, a very well-recognized phenotype.

The prevalence of metabolic syndrome, as reported from several studies, varies widely, particularly according to the race and criteria used. Based on the US Third National Health and Nutrition Examination Survey (NHANES) (1988–1994) and the ATPIII criteria, Ford et al.[11] reported an age-adjusted prevalence of metabolic syndrome of 23.7% in men and women aged 20 years or older. The prevalence increased from 6.7% among participants aged 20 to 29 years, to 43.5% in participants aged 60 to 69 years, and 42.0% in individuals of at least 70 years of age, respectively. Mexican Americans had the highest age-adjusted prevalence of metabolic syndrome (31.9%).

Using the ATPIII criteria, Pollex et al.[12] analyzed data from aboriginal Canadians, reporting that 29.9% of Oji-Cree adults older than 18 years of age and 43.4% of adults older than 34 years of age had metabolic syndrome. In a Mexican population-based survey, the prevalence of metabolic syndrome, according to ATPIII criteria, was 26.6%.[13] In Northwest China the prevalence of metabolic syndrome was 7.9% and 10.8% according to ATPIII and IDF criteria;[14] prevalence increased with age and was higher in women than in men. In Thai adults 35 years and older, using data from a nationally representative sample (the Inter-ASIA study), the prevalence of metabolic syndrome by the IDF and ATPIII criteria were 24.0% (men 16.4%, women 31.6%) and 32.6% (men 28.7%, women 36.4%), respectively.[15] The difference in prevalence between genders was much greater for the IDF compared with the ATPIII definition. Further, the ATPIII definition captures more cases of metabolic syndrome compared with the IDF definition. In Arab Americans, the age-adjusted prevalence of the metabolic syndrome was 23% by ATPIII.[16] The results from these representative population studies show that metabolic syndrome is highly prevalent and may have an important implication for the health-care sector. Thus, the prevention of hypertension and metabolic syndrome should be a public health priority to reduce incidences of cardiovascular diseases.

Since hypomagnesemia is highly related to dyslipidemia, hyperglycemia, and high blood pressure (components of the metabolic syndrome), it appears reasonable to consider them plausible links in the epidemiology of the metabolic syndrome. In this chapter, we review the evidence demonstrating a link between magnesium and the metabolic syndrome.

Possible mechanisms linking hypomagnesemia with metabolic syndrome

Although the underlying mechanisms for many of the pleiotropic effects of magnesium are not well understood, several pathways have been described to explain the link between magnesium and metabolic disorders such as dyslipidemia (hypertriglyceridemia and/or low HDL), hyperglycemia, and high blood pressure.

Magnesium and dyslipidemia

The anti-atherogenic effects of the magnesium profile appear to involve the modification of several enzymes linked with lipid metabolism, inhibiting the activity of lecithin cholesterol acyl transferase (LCAT) and HMG-CoA reductase, and stimulating the activity of lipoprotein lipase.[17] Magnesium is necessary for LCAT's activity, which lowers triglyceride and raises HDL-C levels.[18] Furthermore, the enzyme that deactivates HMG-CoA reductase requires magnesium.[19]

Magnesium and hyperglycemia

Magnesium is involved in more than 300 enzymatic reactions, including glycogen breakdown, fat oxidation, and ATP synthesis.[20] In addition, disorders of intracellular magnesium homeostasis decrease tyrosine kinase activity at insulin receptors, increasing insulin resistance,[21,22] and negatively influence glucose-stimulated insulin secretion,[23] decreasing beta-cell function. Furthermore, low serum magnesium levels are strongly related with elevated serum concentrations of both tumor necrosis factor alpha[24] and C-reactive protein.[25] Magnesium deficiency appears to be involved in the triggering of low-grade inflammatory responses. Through mechanisms related to the increase of insulin resistance, the decrease of insulin secretion, and the triggering of low-grade chronic inflammation syndrome, hypomagnesemia could be involved in the pathogenesis of hyperglycemia.

Magnesium and hypertension

Magnesium inhibits the effects of calcium from vascular smooth muscle sarcoplasmic reticulum by competing for a calcium receptor on a calcium-regulated efflux channel.[26] Furthermore, magnesium attenuates the adverse effects of sodium, stimulating the activity of Na-K ATPase[27] and improving myocardial contractility[28] and endothelium-dependent vasodilation.[29] Finally, magnesium transporters appear to be implicated as a signaling kinase involved in vascular smooth muscle cell growth and apoptosis, processes involved in the vascular remodeling associated with hypertension and other vascular diseases.[30]

An inverse relationship between obesity (as a measure of waist circumference) and serum magnesium levels has been reported,[31] which could be the consequence of the adoption of westernized diets that promote obesity and have declining concentrations of trace elements. Low serum magnesium levels are likely to be an effect rather than a cause of obesity. However, it has been suggested that magnesium could be the cause of obesity, rather than the effect, through a mechanism that involves the interaction of magnesium with fatty acids in the intestine, forming soaps that may reduce the digestible energy content of the diet.[32] In this way, a low intake of magnesium can reduce the forming soap in the intestine, increasing the energy content of the diet. Undoubtedly, further research is needed to test this hypothesis.

Body of evidence

In a cross-sectional population study by Guerrero-Romero et al.[33] of 192 patients of Mexican origin with metabolic syndrome (according to the ATPIII criteria) and 384 matched healthy control subjects, low serum magnesium levels were associated with an elevated risk of metabolic syndrome. The odds ratio (OR) of having the syndrome for those in the lowest quartile of serum magnesium levels was 6.8 (95% CI 4.2–10.9) compared with participants in higher quartiles.[33] Song et al.[34] analyzed data from the Women's Health Study and reported an inverse relationship between dietary intake of magnesium and the prevalence of metabolic syndrome (using ATPIII criteria). Women in the highest quintile of magnesium intake had a lower risk of metabolic syndrome (OR 0.73; 95% CI 0.60–0.88). Using the ATPIII criteria, He et al.[35] prospectively examined the relationship between magnesium intake and incident metabolic syndrome among 4637 Americans aged 18 to 30 years, who were free from metabolic syndrome and diabetes at baseline. Magnesium intake was inversely associated with an incidence of metabolic syndrome. Compared with those in the lowest quartile of magnesium intake, the multivariable-adjusted hazard ratio of metabolic syndrome for participants in the highest quartile was 0.69 (95% CI 0.52–0.91).[35] In a case-control design study, we enrolled incident cases of metabolic syndrome (using ATPIII criteria) that were compared with healthy control subjects, matched by age and gender. Multivariate analysis, adjusted by age, sex, body mass index, waist-to-hip ratio, and total adiposity, showed a strong association between metabolic syndrome and hypomagnesemia (OR 1.9, 95% CI 1.3–7.1). After additional adjustment by C-reactive protein (OR 1.4, 95% CI 1.1–5.9) and malondialdehyde (a lipid peroxidation marker) (OR 1.6, 95% CI 1.1–7.4) levels, metabolic syndrome remained associated with hypomagnesemia, supporting the hypothesis that serum magnesium levels are independently associated with metabolic syndrome.[36]

Using data from NHANES 1988–1994, Ford et al.[37] compared the prevalence of metabolic syndrome (using ATPIII criteria) and daily magnesium intake, and reported an unadjusted prevalence of metabolic syndrome of 29.0% (27.5%, 25.8%, 23.9%, and 21.8%) for the lowest quintile of magnesium intake.[37] The ORs for the second through the fifth quintiles of magnesium intake among all participants were 0.84 (95% CI 0.58–1.23), 0.76 (95% CI 0.54–1.07), 0.62 (95% CI 0.40–0.98), and 0.56 (95% CI 0.34–0.92), respectively; these associations were similar for men and women.

Furthermore, Mirmiran et al.,[38] using ATPIII criteria in Tehran adults, analyzed the association of dietary magnesium intake with metabolic syndrome. After stratifying by age, the association between magnesium intake and metabolic syndrome was significant and not affected by confounders in those individuals aged equal to or greater than 50 years (β –0.11; 95% CI 0.020–0.03, $p < 0.001$). Nonetheless, there was no association between magnesium intake with metabolic syndrome in those individuals aged less than 50 years. In addition, in elderly subjects from Tehran, the overall prevalence of metabolic syndrome (using ATPIII criteria) was 43.8%; individuals with metabolic syndrome exhibited lower serum magnesium levels compared with subjects without the syndrome.[39]

In order to evaluate the association between severe hypomagnesemia and the low-grade inflammatory response in subjects with metabolic syndrome, 98 individuals with a new diagnosis of metabolic syndrome were enrolled in a cross-sectional study. Severe hypomagnesemia (serum magnesium equal to or lower than 1.2 mg/dL), hypomagnesemia (serum magnesium levels greater than 1.2 but less than or equal to 1.8 mg/dL), and normomagnesemia (magnesium levels greater than 1.8 mg/dL) were identified in 21 (21.4%), 38 (38.8%), and 39 (39.8%) individuals, respectively. The ORs, adjusted by waist circumference, showed that severe hypomagnesemia (OR 8.1, 95% CI 3.6–19.4; and OR 3.7, 95% CI 1.1–12.1), but not hypomagnesemia (OR 1.8, 95% CI 0.9–15.5; and OR 1.6, 95% CI 0.7–3.6), was strongly associated with elevated highly sensitive C-reactive protein (hsCRP) and TNF-α levels.[40] These findings support the hypothesis that hypomagnesemia is associated with some aspects of the pathogenesis of metabolic syndrome and plays an important role in triggering a low-grade chronic inflammatory response. Furthermore, it has been observed that magnesium intake, or serum magnesium levels, are associated with all the features of metabolic syndrome.

Conclusion

Evidence about the relationship between magnesium intake and serum levels and metabolic syndrome is derived from observational studies. Results are consistent and there is an inverse association between magnesium intake and/or serum levels and metabolic syndrome. However, no data exists from randomized clinical trials focusing on the prevention or treatment of metabolic syndrome.

According to the IDF's recommendations,[9] the diagnosis of metabolic syndrome requires an uncompromising management strategy that would aim to reduce the risk of cardiovascular disease and type 2 diabetes. To this end, the IDF recommends the primary management of metabolic syndrome through healthy lifestyle promotion strategies: moderate calorie restriction (to achieve a 5%–10% loss of body weight in the first year), a moderate increase in physical activity, and a change in dietary composition. The evidence shows that adequate magnesium intake or a diet rich in magnesium (from whole grains, nuts, green leafy vegetables, dried fruit, and shellfish) may be important for maintaining good cardiometabolic health and is complementary to other healthy lifestyle interventions.[41,42] This would support dietary changes endorsed by the IDF as a preventive or therapeutic strategy against metabolic syndrome.

Further, although oral magnesium supplementation is supported by epidemiological studies, randomized clinical trials are needed to confirm the potential role of magnesium supplementation as a possible public health strategy in the prevention and/or treatment of metabolic syndrome. Until then, the role of magnesium supplementation will remain enigmatic, and thus, the endorsement of dietary magnesium supplements remains unsubstantiated.

References

1. Executive summary of the third report of the National Cholesterol Education Program (NCEP) Expert Panel on Detection, Evaluation, and Treatment of High Blood Cholesterol in Adults (Adult Treatment Panel III). *JAMA* 2001;285:2486–97.
2. Barbagallo M, Dominguez LJ. Magnesium intake in the pathophysiology and treatment of the cardiometabolic syndrome: Where are we in 2006? *J Cardiometab Syndr* 2006;1:356–7.
3. He K, Song Y, Belin RJ, et al. Magnesium intake and metabolic syndrome: Epidemiologic evidence to date. *J Cardiometabol Syndr* 2006;1:351–5.
4. Grundy SM. Metabolic syndrome pandemic. *Arterioscler Thromb Vasc Biol* 2008;28:629–36.
5. Kahn R, Buse J, Ferrannini E, Stern M; American Diabetes Association; European Association for the Study of Diabetes. The metabolic syndrome: Time for a critical appraisal; Joint statement from the American Diabetes Association and the European Association for the Study of Diabetes. *Diabetes Care* 2005;28:2289–304.
6. Gale EA. The myth of the metabolic syndrome. *Diabetologia* 2005;48:1679–83.
7. Bruce KD, Byrne CD. The metabolic syndrome: Common origins of a multifactorial disorder. *Postgrad Med J* 2009;85:614–21.
8. Grundy SM, Cleeman JI, Daniels SR, Donato KA, Eckel RH, Franklin BA, Gordon DJ, et al.; American Heart Association; National Heart, Lung, and Blood Institute. Diagnosis and management of the metabolic syndrome: An American Heart Association/National Heart, Lung, and Blood Institute scientific statement. *Circulation* 2005;112:2735–52.
9. International Diabetes Federation. The IDF consensus worldwide definition of the metabolic syndrome. Brussels: IDF Communication, 2006 (available at: https://www.idf.org/webdata/docs/MetS_def_update2006.pdf).

10. Alberti KG, Zimmet P, Shaw J. The metabolic syndrome: A new worldwide definition. *Lancet* 2005;366:1059–62.
11. Ford ES, Giles WH, Dietz WH. Prevalence of the metabolic syndrome among US adults: Findings from the third National Health and Nutrition Examination Survey. *JAMA* 2002;16287:356–9.
12. Pollex RL, Hanley AJ, Zinman B, Harris SB, Khan HM, Hegele RA. Metabolic syndrome in aboriginal Canadians: Prevalence and genetic associations. *Atherosclerosis* 2006;184:121–9.
13. Aguilar-Salinas CA, Rojas R, Gómez-Pérez FJ, Mehta R, Franco A, Olaiz G, Rull JA. The metabolic syndrome: A concept hard to define. *Arch Med Res* 2005;36:223–31.
14. Zhao Y, Yan H, Yang R, Li Q, Dang S, Wang Y. Prevalence and determinants of metabolic syndrome among adults in a rural area of Northwest China. *PLoS One* 2014;9:e91578.
15. Aekplakorn W, Chongsuvivatwong V, Tatsanavivat P, Suriyawongpaisal P. Prevalence of metabolic syndrome defined by the International Diabetes Federation and National Cholesterol Education Program criteria among Thai adults. *Asia Pac J Public Health* 2011;23:792–800.
16. Jaber LA, Brown MB, Hammad A, Zhu Q, Herman WH. The prevalence of the metabolic syndrome among Arab Americans. *Diabetes Care* 2004;27:234–8.
17. Belin RJ, He K. Magnesium physiology and pathogenic mechanisms that contribute to the development of the metabolic syndrome. *Magnes Res* 2007;20:107–29.
18. Touyz RM, Panz V, Milne FJ. Relations between magnesium, calcium, and plasma renin activity in black and white hypertensive patients. *Miner Electrolyte Metab* 1995;21:417–22.
19. Field FJ, Henning B, Mathur SN. In vitro regulation of 3-hydroxy-3-methyl-glutarylcoenzyme A reductase and acylcoenzyme A: Cholesterol acyltrans-ferase activities by phosphorylation-dephosphorylation in rabbit intestine. *Biochim Biophys Acta* 1984;802:9–16.
20. Lukaski HC. Magnesium, zinc, and chromium nutriture and physical activity. *Am J Clin Nutr* 2000;72:585S–93S.
21. Suarez A, Pulido N, Casla A, et al. Impaired tyrosine-kinase activity of muscle insulin receptors from hypomagnesaemic rats. *Diabetologia* 1995;38:1262–70.
22. Paolisso G, Barbagallo M. Hypertension, diabetes mellitus, and insulin resistance: The role of intracellular magnesium. *Am J Hypertens* 1997;10:346–55.
23. Barbagallo M, Dominguez LJ, Galioto A, et al. Role of magnesium in insulin action, diabetes and cardio-metabolic syndrome X. *Mol Aspects Med* 2003;24:39–52.
24. Rodríguez-Morán M, Guerrero-Romero F. Elevated serum concentration of tumor necrosis factor-alpha is linked to low serum magnesium levels in the obesity-related inflammatory response. *Magnes Res* 2004;17:189–96.
25. Guerrero-Romero F, Rodríguez-Morán M. Relationship between serum magnesium levels and C-reactive protein concentration, in non-diabetic, non-hypertensive obese subjects. *Int J Obes Relat Metab Disord* 2002;26:469–74.
26. Stephenson EW, Podolsky RJ. Regulation by magnesium of intracellular calcium movement in skinned muscle fibers. *J Gen Physiol* 1977;69:1–16.
27. Touyz RM. Role of magnesium in the pathogenesis of hypertension. *Mol Aspects Med* 2003;24:107–36.

28. Chakraborti S, Chakraborti T, Mandal M, et al. Protective role of magnesium in cardiovascular diseases: A review. *Mol Cell Biochem* 2002;238:163–79.
29. Pearson PJ, Evora PR, Seccombe JF, et al. Hypomagnesemia inhibits nitric oxide release from coronary endothelium: Protective role of magnesium infusion after cardiac operations. *Ann Thorac Surg* 1998;65:967–72.
30. Touyz RM. Transient receptor potential melastatin 6 and 7 channels, magnesium transport and vascular biology: Implications in hypertension. *Am J Physiol Heart Circ Physiol* 2008;294:H1103–18.
31. Drenick EJ. The influence of ingestion of calcium and other soap-forming substances on fecal fat. *Gastroenterology.* 1961;41:242–44.
32. Huang JH, Lu YF, Cheng FC, Lee JN, Tsai LC. Correlation of magnesium intake with metabolic parameters, depression and physical activity in elderly type 2 diabetes patients: A cross-sectional study. *Nutr J* 2012;11:41.
33. Guerrero-Romero F, Rodriguez-Moran M. Low serum magnesium levels and metabolic syndrome. *Acta Diabetol* 2002;39:209–13.
34. Song Y, Ridker PM, Manson JE, Cook NR, Buring JE, Liu S. Magnesium intake, C-reactive protein, and the prevalence of metabolic syndrome in middle-aged and older U.S. women. *Diabetes Care* 2005;28:1438–44.
35. He K, Liu K, Daviglus ML, Morris SJ, Loria CM, Van Horn L, Jacobs DR Jr, Savage PJ. Magnesium intake and incidence of metabolic syndrome among young adults. *Circulation* 2006;113:1675–82.
36. Guerrero-Romero F, Rodríguez-Morán M. Hypomagnesemia, oxidative stress, inflammation, and metabolic syndrome. *Diabetes Metab Res Rev* 2006;22:471–6.
37. Ford ES, Li C, McGuire LC, Mokdad AH, Liu S. Intake of dietary magnesium and the prevalence of the metabolic syndrome among U.S. adults. *Obesity (Silver Spring)* 2007;15:1139–46.
38. Mirmiran P, Shab-Bidar S, Hosseini-Esfahani F, Asghari G, Hosseinpour-Niazi S, Azizi F. Magnesium intake and prevalence of metabolic syndrome in adults: Tehran Lipid and Glucose Study. *Public Health Nutr* 2012;15:693–701.
39. Ghasemi A, Zahediasl S, Syedmoradi L, Azizi F. Low serum magnesium levels in elderly subjects with metabolic syndrome. *Biol Trace Elem Res.*2010;136:18–25.
40. Guerrero-Romero F, Bermudez-Peña C, Rodriguez-Moran M. Severe hypomagnesemia and low-grade inflammation in metabolic syndrome. *Magnes Res* 2011;24:45–53.
41. Gums JG. Magnesium in cardiovascular and other disorders. *Am J Health-Syst Pharm* 2004;61:1569–76.
42. Saris NE, Mervaala E, Karppanen H, Khawaja JA, Lewenstam A. Magnesium: An update on physiological, clinical and analytical aspects. *Clin Chem Acta* 2000;294:1–26.

chapter seven

Low magnesium plays a central role in high blood pressure

Andrea Rosanoff

Contents

Abbreviations

CLMD   chronic latent magnesium deficit
DASH   Dietary Approaches to Stop Hypertension
HDL   high-density lipoprotein
LDL   low-density lipoprotein
Mg   magnesium
TOPH   Trials of Hypertension Prevention
UNaV   urinary sodium excretion

Introduction

Magnesium (Mg) has direct and indirect effects on blood pressure, both of which are substantial. Directly, Mg causes blood vessels to relax and dilate, which is necessary for normal blood pressure. Indirectly, proper Mg status allows the cellular balance, transport, and utilization of other "electrolytes" such as sodium, potassium, and calcium. Low potassium alone can cause high blood pressure. However, even adequate potassium cannot normalize high blood pressure if Mg in the blood is too low. Adequate Mg and potassium are required to maintain normal blood pressure. Given the low nutritional intakes of both Mg and potassium in the United States, it is not surprising that 30.4% of U.S. adults have high blood pressure,[1] which is a major risk factor for early death and cardiovascular diseases.

Hypertension is associated with stroke and heart disease and continually strains the heart, blood vessels, and kidneys. Hypertension is referred to as the "silent killer," because it may often go unnoticed, even over the span of years.[2] In 2013, about 77.9 million U.S. adults had hypertension.[3] The incidence of hypertension continues to rise. From 1999 to 2009, high blood pressure among the U.S. population rose by 17.1% and deaths attributed to hypertension rose by 43.6%.[3] Consumption of a mostly "Western diet," which comprises processed foods that are generally low in both Mg and potassium, may contribute to difficulty in controlling hypertension.[4-6] Physicians can play an important role in helping their patients prevent and treat high blood pressure, and knowledge of Mg research in this area is key to the success of both.

Preventing and treating high blood pressure means good micronutrient nutrition

Magnesium challenges high blood pressure

A 2009 study among emergency room patients showed intravenous Mg sulfate therapy to be as effective as anti-hypertensive medications at lowering blood pressure.[7] One recent meta-analysis on subjects with very high blood pressure (systolic blood pressure >155 mmHg at baseline) showed highly significant reductions in both systolic and diastolic blood pressure with oral Mg therapy, comparable to those found with anti-hypertensive medications.[8] However, between 1983 and 2014, several randomized controlled trials tested oral Mg supplements in the treatment of mostly mild hypertensive and/or normotensive subjects, with seriously conflicting results. Four meta-analyses using various sets of these studies have all demonstrated statistically significant but clinically small changes (or no change) in blood pressure with Mg supplementation.[9-12] Such conflicting and seemingly minimal results have made oral Mg supplementation for hypertension a hard sell to physicians and medical providers. Let's explore these studies carefully.

Findings from "magnesium for hypertension" research

1. Impact of magnesium dose
Of the 47 published articles[13-59] reporting 49 studies of oral Mg therapy for hypertension performed between 1983 and 2014 (see Table 7.1), 30 studies[13-23,31-38,42-52] tested doses of Mg between 120 and 394 mg/day, which are below the recommended daily allowance (RDA) for adult men (400–420 mg Mg/day; 16.5–17.3 mmol Mg/day). Eight of these 49 studies[13,14,32,33,42-45] administered Mg doses below the RDA for adult women (310–320 mg Mg/day; 12.8–13.1 mmol Mg/day). The RDA is the amount of a nutrient necessary to maintain health in 97.5% of the healthy population, not the presumably higher amount needed to achieve health for unhealthy individuals.

Table 7.1 Summary of Mg supplement studies for blood pressure, 1983–2014

Study citation	Mg dose, mg/day	Form of Mg	BP status at baseline, NT or HT	Medical status at baseline, T or UT	BP outcome	Notes
Borrello et al.[13]	120	MgO	HT	UT	No change	Drop in SBP only
Nowson and Morgan[14]	240	Aspartate	HT	UT	No change	
Ferrara et al.[15]	365	Pidolate	HT	UT	No change	
Lind et al.[16]	365	Lactate and citrate	HT	UT	No change	
de Valk et al.[17]	365	Aspartate HCl	HT	UT	No change	
Plum-Wirell et al.[18]	365	Aspartate	HT	UT	No change	
Wirell et al.[19]	365	Aspartate	HT	UT	No change	
Cappuccio et al.[20]	365	Aspartate	HT	UT	No change (decrease in DBP only)	
Reyes et al.[21]	384	$MgCl_2$	HT	UT	No change (decrease in DBP only)	Medication interrupted 2–3 mo pre-study
Olhaberry et al.[22]	384	$MgCl_2$	HT	UT	No change (decrease in SBP only)	Medication interrupted 4 wk pre-study
Purvis et al.[23]	389	$MgCl_2$	HT	UT	No change (decrease in SBP only)	

(Continued)

Table 7.1 (Continued) Summary of Mg supplement studies for blood pressure, 1983–2014

Study citation	Mg dose, mg/day	Form of Mg	BP status at baseline, NT or HT	Medical status at baseline, T or UT	BP outcome	Notes
Witteman et al.[24]	486	Aspartate HCl	HT	UT	No change (decrease in DBP only)	With 2,340 mg/day potassium supplement
Patki et al.[25]	486	MgCl₂	HT	UT	Decrease	
Walker et al.[26]	607	Amino acid chelate	HT	UT	No change	Mg replete subjects
Haga[27]	607	MgO	HT	UT	Decrease	MBP measured
Motoyama et al.[28]	607	MgO	HT	UT	Decrease	No medications during study or 1 mo pre-study, at least
Sanjuliani et al.[29]	607	MgO	HT	UT	Decrease	No medications 2 wk pre-study or during study
Zemel et al.[30]	972	Aspartate	HT	UT	No change	Mg replete subjects
Widman et al.[31]	365	Mg(OH)₂	HT	UT	No change	
	972	Mg(OH)₂	HT	UT	Decrease	
Shafique et al.[32]	240	MgCl₂	HT	T	Decrease	
Sebekova et al.[33]	255	Aspartate HCl	HT	T	Decrease	Interrupted medications

(Continued)

Table 7.1 (Continued) Summary of Mg supplement studies for blood pressure, 1983–2014

Study citation	Mg dose, mg/day	Form of Mg	BP status at baseline, NT or HT	Medical status at baseline, T or UT	BP outcome	Notes
Michon[34]	323	Slow-mag/B_6	HT	T	Decrease	
Wirell et al.[35]	365	Aspartate	HT	T	Decrease	
Dyckner and Wester[36]	365	Aspartate HCl	HT	T	Decrease	Beta-blockers
Rodriguez-Moran and Guerrero-Romero[37]	381	$MgCl_2$	HT	T	Decrease	Pre-diabetic with low serum Mg
Paolisso et al.[38]	384	Pidolate	HT	T	Decrease	
Guerrero-Romero and Rodriguez-Moran[39]	450	$MgCl_2$	HT	T	Decrease	
Kawano et al.[40]	486	MgO	HT	T	Decrease	
Saito et al.[41]	607	MgO	50% HT 50% NT	T	Decrease	
Doyle et al.[42]	250	$Mg(OH)_2$	NT	UT	No change	
Lee et al.[43]	300	MgO	NT	Unknown	No change	
Henderson et al.[44]	304	MgO	NT	T	No change	
Guerrero-Romero et al.[45]	304	MgCl2	NT	UT	No change	
Sacks et al.[46]	340	Lactate	NT	UT	No change	
TOHP Study Group[47]	365	Diglycine	NT	UT	No change	
Mooren et al.[48]	365	Aspartate HCl	NT	Not reported	No change	
Sibai et al.[49]	365	Aspartate HCl	NT	UT	No change	Pregnancy

(Continued)

Table 7.1 (Continued) Summary of Mg supplement studies for blood pressure, 1983–2014

Study citation	Mg dose, mg/day	Form of Mg	BP status at baseline, NT or HT	Medical status at baseline, T or UT	BP outcome	Notes
Sacks et al.[50]	365	Diglycine chelate	NT	UT	No change	Given with Ca or K
Simental-Mendia et al.[51]	382	MgCl$_2$	NT	UT	No change	
Cosaro et al.[52]	394	Pidolate	NT	UT	No change	
Itoh et al.[53]	413–583	Mg(OH)2	NT	Some treated "when necessary"	Decrease	Baseline statistics may be faulty
Rodriguez-Moran and Guerrero-Romero[54]	450	MgCl$_2$	Borderline HT/NT	T	No change	
Rodriguez-Hernandez et al.[55]	450	MgCl$_2$	NT	UT	No change	
Daly et al.[56]	500	MgO	NT	UT	No change	
Kisters et al.[57]	505	Aspartate	NT	UT	No change	
Warry et al.[58]	600	Lactate + B$_6$	NT	UT	No change	
Guerrero-Romero and Rodriguez-Moran[59]	632	MgCl$_2$	NT	UT	Decrease	Subjects had low serum Mg
Mean Mg dose (range), mg/day	430 (120–972)					

Findings: (1) Untreated hypertensive patients need higher doses of oral Mg ($\geq$600 mg/day) than treated hypertensive patients to lower blood pressure. (2) Oral Mg, even at a high dose (i.e., $\geq$600 mg/day), does not decrease blood pressure in normotensive patients. (3) Oral Mg therapy does not decrease blood pressure in Mg-replete hypertensive patients; potassium supplements may do so.

Abbreviations: DBP, diastolic BP; HT, hypertensive at baseline (60% of studies); NT, normotensive at baseline (40% of studies); SBP, systolic BP; T, most or all subjects treated with anti-hypertensive medications (30% of studies); TOHP, Trials of Hypertension Prevention; UT, untreated, in which most or all subjects not treated with anti-hypertensive medications (70% of studies).

Because hypertension is not part of a healthy state, it makes sense for studies on high blood pressure to try Mg doses higher than the RDA.

For most unmedicated patients presenting with essential hypertension, oral Mg therapy of at least 486 mg Mg/day along with 2340 mg/day potassium supplementation was necessary to show a significant decrease in both systolic and diastolic blood pressure[25] (see Table 7.1). Only when doses of ≥600 mg Mg/day were tested did a majority (four out of six) of such studies on unmedicated hypertensive subjects show oral Mg's ability to significantly lower both systolic and diastolic blood pressure;[27-29,31] the remaining two studies in this category failed to show any significant change in blood pressure but were both deemed "Mg replete" by the studies' authors (see below) (see Table 7.1).[26,30] Furthermore, in the one publication with Mg for hypertension that used escalating doses of Mg, investigators found that Mg did not reduce high blood pressure in these unmedicated hypertensives with a 365 mg/day Mg dose, whereas a significant decrease in blood pressure was achieved with 720 mg/day Mg.[31] Oral Mg therapy for hypertensive patients already using anti-hypertensive medications is effective at much smaller daily doses of oral Mg therapy (i.e., as little as 240 mg Mg/day; see Table 7.1). Thus, careful analysis of these randomized controlled trials shows that several studies used a Mg dose that was too low to show a significant effect on high blood pressure, and that subjects taking anti-hypertensive medications react differently to Mg supplementation than non-medicated subjects.

2. Impact of hypertension status

Blood pressure medications "lower" blood pressure, whereas proper Mg micronutrient supplementation has the ability to "normalize" it. Even so, many studies seem to make a point of reporting that Mg does not lower normal blood pressure. We would not expect nor desire Mg supplements to cause "low blood pressure" in normotensive patients. Of 49 studies of oral Mg therapy for hypertension conducted between 1983 and 2014, 39% (n = 19 studies) were conducted on subjects with normal blood pressure (i.e., ≤140/90 mmHg) (Table 7.1).[41-59] This may explain why the overall results of these studies in meta-analyses showed a minimal clinical effect of oral Mg for hypertension.[9-12] The one meta-analysis that included only studies with high starting systolic blood pressure, in contrast, showed large clinically relevant decreases in both systolic and diastolic blood pressure with Mg supplementation that were statistically significant.[8] The largest single study on oral Mg therapy and blood pressure thus far is the Trials of Hypertension Prevention (TOPH) study,[47] done on a large sample (n = 227) of normotensive subjects. These healthy subjects showed no change in blood pressure after 6 months with oral Mg therapy. In reality, the TOPH study was testing whether Mg supplementation acts like blood pressure medications that lower blood pressure, normal or not. Whereas a dose of blood pressure medication can cause a temporarily low blood pressure in a healthy individual, a dose of oral Mg will not lower a normal, healthy blood pressure. If a person takes in more Mg than necessary, the body will absorb and use what it needs and excrete any excess. The TOPH study used a daily dose of 360 mg, which is not enough to lower a high blood pressure in non-medicated subjects (see above), and all TOPH subjects were healthy, had not taken any medications for at least 2 months, and had normal blood pressure at study initiation. These studies demonstrate that study interpretation and design must be carefully evaluated before valid conclusions can be made.

3. Impact of anti-hypertensive medication usage

Anti-hypertensive medications decrease the Mg dose necessary to significantly lower a high blood pressure.[60] This appears to be true for beta-blockers, angiotensin-converting enzyme inhibitors, and calcium channel blockers, which have all been shown to "spare" or conserve Mg[61,62] by decreasing Mg in the urine.[63-65] Specifically, these anti-hypertensive drugs conserve serum,[66-68] lymphocyte,[69] and intracellular Mg.[70] Long-term use of thiazide diuretics also appears to lower the oral Mg dose necessary to lower high blood pressure (Table 7.1),[60] although the use of these diuretics can result in Mg (as well as potassium) loss through the kidneys.[71]

Mg exhibits properties of a beta-blocker, vasodilator, and calcium channel blocker. When oral Mg therapy is given to hypertensive patients, urinary sodium excretion (UNaV) has been shown to increase,[16,18,53] thus giving Mg some aspects of a natural diuretic as well. Whereas a drug generally acts selectively (usually at one channel or site), Mg acts in all of the organs plus types of membrane channels and sites in vascular smooth muscle that monitor blood pressure. Mg is central to regulation and control of blood vessel contraction and relaxation.[72] Proper calcium:Mg balance allows blood vessel muscles to relax and keeps the heart from over-responding to nerve or hormonal stimulation.[73] Adequate Mg status is the best way to achieve these proper functions, and anti-hypertensive medications can sometimes mask the symptoms of Mg deficiency without replenishing Mg. Some anti-hypertensive medications make Mg deficiency worse by increasing Mg loss in urine.

4. Impact of magnesium status

As mentioned above, all but two studies on unmedicated hypertensives using ≥600 mg Mg/day decreased high blood pressure, but there were two studies in which hypertensive subjects who received such high and even higher doses of Mg did not show a change in high blood pressure.[26,30] These studies both speculated that their test subjects were already "replete" in their Mg status. In such cases, oral Mg therapy as high as 960 mg/day could not alleviate high blood pressure.[30] This shows that

Mg may not be the only micronutrient essential to normal healthy blood pressure. Low potassium can also be a factor. If a patient is replete in Mg and still has high blood pressure, perhaps balancing potassium to sodium status will help normalize the patient's blood pressure without adding anti-hypertensive medications. When the hypertension is due to something other than low Mg status, Mg supplements will not normalize the blood pressure.

Potassium challenges high blood pressure

1. Low potassium plus high salt intake can induce high blood pressure

It is widely held that high blood pressure is caused by high salt (sodium chloride) intakes. However, research shows a higher importance of low potassium intake as well as low potassium:sodium in the etiology of mild to moderate essential hypertension. Before 1900, humans lived in a low-sodium, high-potassium environment; whole grains, fruits, and vegetables appeared at every meal and highly processed foods were non-existent. Our kidneys bear the evidence of our low-sodium/high-potassium environmental history in that they actually store sodium while letting potassium pass in the urine. The average kidney can slow sodium loss to 10 mg/day if it is in short supply. However, the daily minimum potassium loss can be as high as 240 mg, which is 24 times that of sodium. Currently, 94% to >97% of the U.S. population consumes below the adequate intake for potassium, whereas >97% consumes more than the adequate intake of sodium (Table 7.2).[74]

When the sodium:potassium ratio is excessive, the human body tries to eliminate the excess sodium via the sodium-conserving kidneys. With high blood pressure, the kidneys can filter more electrolytes and thus maximize their limited ability to release sodium. Unfortunately, this extra blood processing excretes more potassium, because the kidney does not

Table 7.2 Changes in sodium and potassium intakes in the United States, 1900–2000

	1900	2000
Rate of hypertension	Low	High
Sodium, mg/day	200	5000
Potassium, mg/day	6000	2000
Sodium:potassium ratio	1:30	2.5:1

This table shows the change in average mineral intake and balance that occurred in the U.S. population between 1900 and 2000. Note the great rise in sodium and the decline in potassium intakes plus the rise in incidence of high blood pressure. During the same period, average Mg intake also decreased (Seelig and Rosanoff,[114] p. 61).

naturally conserve potassium. Restricting sodium intake can lower the dietary sodium:potassium ratio. Supplementing potassium in the diet using a half-sodium/half-potassium condiment or salt substitute can help stabilize the sodium:potassium ratio. But a diet consistently high in fruits, vegetables, nuts, legumes, low-fat dairy, and whole grains, such as the DASH diet[75-77] or other similar diets, can provide the sodium:potassium ratio as well as Mg intake that enables normal, healthy blood pressure.

2. Potassium and hypertension

In 1928, decades before the advent of anti-hypertensive medications, Dr. W. L. T. Addison, a practicing physician in Toronto, Canada, showed that potassium lowers blood pressure and sodium raises it. Whenever Addison administered sodium salt, blood pressure increased; administration of potassium salt lowered blood pressure.[78] To make sure that chloride was not influencing the results, Addison repeated the experiment using potassium and sodium bromide and he got the same results. In the early 1930s, another Canadian researcher, W. W. Priddle, lowered the high blood pressure of 100% of his 45 subjects with a combination therapy of low-sodium diet and potassium citrate supplements containing 1685–8295 mg potassium per day.[79] Other studies have shown potassium to lower a high blood pressure while having no effect on normal blood pressure.[80,81]

3. Potassium needs adequate magnesium to regulate blood pressure

Early nutrition studies in humans showed that a Mg deficiency lowered potassium in the blood even when potassium intake was high and sodium in the blood was normal or raised.[82] These two trends yielded a higher blood sodium:potassium ratio even when potassium and sodium intakes were normal. Low Mg status made adequate amounts of potassium unavailable in the body. When the Mg depletion was corrected, however, the potassium status also normalized. Oral Mg supplementation in hypertensive patients has been shown to reduce erythrocyte[38] and plasma sodium,[27] increase UnaV,[16,53] and increase erythrocyte potassium and Mg.[38] Increasing potassium and Mg intake while reducing sodium consumption can potentially ameliorate hypertension in most patients with essential hypertension who live in our modern processed food diet culture. A high-vegetable diet or a DASH-type diet can achieve these dietary levels of low sodium, high potassium, and high Mg, but such diets are difficult for patients to maintain.[83]

Magnesium and calcium

A low Mg status impairs proper calcium metabolism, affecting blood pressure and cardiovascular health. When cells' natural calcium channel blocker, Mg, becomes deficient, calcium will rush abnormally into cells.[84,85] Many aspects of the rise in intracellular calcium ion concentration and its impact on hypertension have been elucidated at the cellular level.[86-90] In itself, a rise in intracellular calcium ions due primarily to a Mg deficiency creates a cellular calcium:Mg imbalance; in the case of vascular smooth muscle cells, this imbalance instills a perpetually high calcium ion level, causing hypertension.[85] In neurons, healthy intracellular Mg ion concentrations block N-type calcium channels at nerve endings, thus inhibiting norepinephrine release and maintaining normal blood pressure.[91] When intracellular Mg is low in these cells, the calcium channels can become unblocked and epinephrine release occurs, causing vasoconstriction and blood pressure elevation. Long-term normal blood pressure requires maintaining healthy calcium and potassium levels, which, in turn, both require adequate cellular Mg. Similar to potassium physiology, when Mg status is low enough to exhibit hypomagnesemia, serum calcium can drop below normal regardless of the intake of calcium,[82] and only the ingestion of Mg in adequate amounts can correct the hypocalcemia.

Resnick et al.[73] showed that the intracellular calcium:Mg ratio is a crucial factor in the etiology of hypertension and other aspects of metabolic syndrome. Resnick's work shows that calcium:Mg cellular ratios above a certain level result in hyperinsulinemia, insulin resistance, platelet aggregation, cardiac hypertrophy, and hypertension. Confirming this finding, Kisters et al.[92] reported that aortic smooth muscle cells of spontaneously hypertensive rats have a calcium:Mg ratio of 3.5 compared with only 2.2 for normal rats.

Anti-hypertensive medications: Lowering blood pressure without magnesium and/or potassium repletion

The current medical approach focuses on medications lowering blood pressure. This approach intends to remove a major risk factor (i.e., high blood pressure) for heart disease and stroke but does not address chronically low intakes of Mg and potassium in the population at large. While anti-hypertensive medications may be necessary to stabilize a very high blood pressure, consumption of Mg and potassium-rich foods and Mg supplementation may be warranted and can be used as either preventive, adjunctive, or monotherapy for many patients. Physicians often promote diet/lifestyle change and exercise as the first course of therapy when a patient presents with elevated blood pressure in the office. In most healthy patients, dietary modification to include Mg and potassium-rich foods can be initiated. However, these diets have been found to be difficult to maintain,[83] and in such cases, Mg (and perhaps potassium) supplementation should be initiated. Blood pressure should be monitored regularly, and physicians and patients should discuss raising the supplement dose at 6 weeks if lower blood pressure is not achieved: if normal blood pressure levels are not adequately achieved by 3–6 months of diet and Mg supplementation, potassium supplements and/or adding prescription anti-hypertensives should be considered. Starting with this adjunctive holistic approach for most patients who are otherwise healthy may help with patient compliance and may be healthier and more economical than anti-hypertensive medication therapies in the long run.

Dietary changes for hypertension

The most common dietary modification suggested by physicians for hypertension is to reduce sodium chloride intake, but Mg and potassium intakes should not be neglected. For otherwise healthy individuals with normal renal function, raising Mg and potassium intakes with supplements is recommended. However, the DASH diet and other healthy food plans can better ensure adequate and balanced amounts of all 44 nutrients essential to humans in addition to healthy levels of potassium, sodium, calcium, and Mg.

Does weight loss improve hypertension?

When patients initiate a weight loss diet by increasing their intake of fruits, vegetables, and whole grains while lowering their saturated fat intake, they are essentially increasing both their potassium and Mg intakes while lowering their requirement for Mg (saturated fat ingestion can substantially increase Mg requirement).[93] For people on such weight-reduction diets, there may be enough change in Mg and potassium status to normalize high blood pressure and potentially reduce other cardiovascular risk factors.

Is salt restriction safer than medications?

The association between sodium intake and elevated blood pressure has been noted since before 1980; however, many medical professionals are cautious about recommending severely salt-restricted diets because sodium is an important essential nutrient, and hyponatremia must be avoided. Alderman and Lamport showed that moderate salt restriction resulted in *elevated* blood pressure for 15% of patients.[94] The study further displayed disturbed sleep patterns with sodium restriction. Other studies showed that salt-restricted diets can increase low-density lipoprotein (LDL) cholesterol.[95] Because most nutritional sodium is derived from grains, dairy, and meats, restriction of these food groups not only lowers sodium but simultaneously reduces the amounts of calcium, iron, Mg, and vitamin B_6 also found in these foods. It is interesting to note that an association has been shown between low-salt diets and an increased risk of heart attack[96] and myocardial infarction in men consuming salt-restricted diets. In men, age- and race-adjusted myocardial infarction incidence in the lowest versus highest 24-hour quartile was 11.5 versus 2.5 (relative risk, 4.3; 95% confidence interval, 1.7–10.6).[97] This may seem a surprising result until one recalls that low sodium excretion goes along with a salt-restricted low Mg diet, and Mg supplementation increases sodium excretion.[16,53] McCarron[98] noted that "when adults meet or exceed the recommended dietary allowances of calcium, potassium, and Mg, the simultaneous ingestion of a diet high in sodium chloride is not associated with elevated arterial pressure. In fact, a higher sodium chloride intake in these adults is most likely associated with the lowest blood pressure in the society."

Salt serves as a preservative, and many traditional processes derive salt from the sea. If the process includes total evaporation, this resource would not be pure sodium chloride, but rather a salt containing all the minerals of the sea, including Mg and potassium. Sodium appears to be the only nutrient that, when low, actually generates a craving.[99] Sodium deprivation alters taste response.[99] Humans require a minimum of 500 mg sodium daily, with the prospect of hyponatremia serving as an important health concern.[100]

The association between salt and hypertension is multifaceted and includes the intakes of Mg and potassium in addition to sodium. For blood pressure control, sodium and potassium require a ratio in which sodium is not too high, and Mg must be adequate. If Mg and potassium are adequate, an individual is highly unlikely to experience essential hypertension.[98] Nevertheless, even with proper sodium and potassium balance, low Mg can result in an increased intracellular calcium:Mg ratio and a subsequent increase in blood pressure.[73] When Mg status is healthy and cellular Mg balances well with calcium, a low intake of potassium coupled with high salt can cause essential hypertension that is not associated with metabolic syndrome. As such, all four electrolyte minerals are important in blood pressure health.

Hypertension can be corrected by Mg (see Table 7.1) and/or potassium repletion[80] in many individuals.[81] Healthy individuals with an adequate supply of dietary Mg show low rates of hypertension;[81,101,102] when both Mg and potassium are adequate, healthy people are able to tolerate a high-salt diet, especially if their calcium:Mg status is balanced. In fact, a review of observational data from several large databases shows that a high sodium chloride intake in these adults is most likely associated with the lowest blood pressure in society.[81,98,101]

Putting magnesium to work for your patients

Warning: Any patient with kidney disease (renal failure) must be evaluated closely and continuously when either Mg and/or potassium supplements are prescribed.

Preventing hypertension in your healthy patients

Patients can best maintain their healthy blood pressure with a diet adequate or even high in nutritional Mg and potassium, two essential nutrients that are quite low in usual modern diets.[103] The Dietary Approaches to Stop Hypertension (DASH) diet[104] has been shown to contain 500 mg Mg/day, whereas the usual processed food diet has only 160 mg Mg.[105] In addition, the DASH diet also raises calcium and potassium intakes while lowering sodium intake (see Table 7.2).[105] The DASH diet provides adequate Mg and potassium nutrition; however, the calcium:Mg ratio, while lower than usual diets, is still above the recommended level of 2.0. Decreasing dairy by replacing 1 cup of dairy per day with 1.3 oz of nuts in the DASH diet will lower the calcium:Mg ratio to a safe level (<2.0) while delivering the same amount of calories per day. Vegetarian diets coupled with meditation[106,107] provide proper Mg and potassium nutrition and lower the Mg requirement by decreasing the stress response.[108] The Mediterranean Diet[109] is high in fiber, Mg, and potassium due to its high content of fruits, vegetables, nuts, seeds, and whole grains. Unfortunately, these dietary and lifestyle approaches toward hypertension treatment are not consistently achievable for all patients.[76] For such people, nutritional supplements are a viable option. For people with healthy blood pressure, oral Mg therapy at doses of 100–400 mg Mg/day should suffice. However, attaining adequate potassium in a supplement form is difficult, because most potassium supplements are 99 mg potassium/pill, requiring 47 pills to equal 1 day's intake of potassium from the DASH diet.

Physicians' steps to healthier blood pressure

1. Determine if your patients with hypertension have primary or secondary hypertension

Secondary hypertension is a less common but important cause of hypertension and should be ruled out as an initial step in the hypertension workup. Normalizing blood pressure in these individuals may be achieved by treating the causing factor (tumor, kidney disease, or other diagnosis). The following discussion concerns primary or essential hypertension.

2. Determine if your patient has mild, moderate,
severe, or refractory hypertension. Does the
patient have metabolic syndrome?

The severity of hypertension must dictate the treatment program. If blood pressure is dangerously high, immediate drug therapy is very important while you help your patient make long-term changes in Mg, calcium:Mg, and potassium status. For those with moderate hypertension or pre-hypertension, oral Mg therapy (at levels of at least 600 mg/day Mg[27-29,31] or 480 mg/day Mg plus 2340 mg/day potassium[25]) is definitely worth trying before prescribing diuretics or other anti-hypertensive medications. It should be noted that caution should be used in chronic kidney disease patients. Blood pressure should be rechecked, ideally, at three separate office visits after about 6–8 weeks of initiating Mg supplementation in order to ensure efficacy or to change the treatment modality or dose. As with medications, monitoring patients' adherence to the supplementation program as well as their blood pressure is essential. Some patients respond well to this level of oral Mg therapy, whereas others experience gastrointestinal side effects including diarrhea or uncomfortably soft stools. These side effects can be overcome by spreading the Mg dose administration from one to two or three times per day, changing the prescription from Mg oxide to one of Mg's chelated forms, or lowering the oral Mg dose while adding a transdermal Mg application, ideally twice daily.[110] In addition, some patients may do well on the DASH or Ornish dietary programs mentioned above if their hypertension is moderate or mild and their dedication to diet/lifestyle changes is high.

If a patient's hypertension is part of a larger metabolic syndrome (i.e., the blood glucose parameters are also high), the patient will likely exhibit a high intracellular calcium:Mg ratio.[73] Risk factors for metabolic syndrome include low high-density lipoprotein (HDL) cholesterol, hyperglycemia, and central abdominal obesity. The presence of these symptoms yields a high suspicion for the diagnosis of this syndrome, and such patients can benefit from oral Mg therapy. If aspects of metabolic syndrome are not present, the hypertensive patient may have adequate Mg status but a low potassium intake that is causing the high blood pressure. The DASH diet and/or switching to a potassium-containing salt that also lowers sodium intake may prove beneficial. Always keep in mind that adequate Mg is necessary to utilize potassium and calcium properly and that hypertension and hypomagnesemia can both or either manifest without any other symptoms of metabolic syndrome. Check for calcium intake and supplement use: strive for a calcium:Mg intake of 2.0 (weight to weight) in addition to Mg adequacy for long-term health.

3. Assess your patient's medications

Evaluation of patient medication is important prior to supplementation, and changes to medications should be considered if medically acceptable. For example, for patients taking potassium-sparing diuretics such as triamterene (Maxzide and Dyazide) or spironolactone (Aldactone), physicians may consider a replacement medication prior to potassium supplementation. If patients continue to take such medications, their plasma potassium should be monitored closely to ensure that it does not become dangerously high. In addition, beta-blockers reduce the control of plasma potassium during potassium loading. Physicians should consider changing this medication prior to potassium supplementation. Thiazide diuretics can cause potassium and Mg loss, rendering replenishment of potassium and Mg difficult. Finally, proton pump inhibitors can trigger hypomagnesemia as a side effect. Assessing acceptable alternative medications when possible is encouraged.

For hypertensive patients not taking any anti-hypertensive medications, the initial Mg oral dose should be ≥600 mg/day. For patients taking anti-hypertensive medication for at least 6 months, the Mg dose to lower blood pressure can be lower (i.e., 240–450 mg/day).[60] It should be noted that caution is advised in chronic kidney disease patients.

4. If possible, obtain baseline serum potassium and magnesium values

Serum potassium tends to reflect total body potassium, serving as a potential benchmark by which to assess a patient's therapy program. In cases of baseline hypokalemia (potassium <4 mEq/l), a patient's potassium should be re-evaluated every 2–3 weeks until it is in the range of 4–5 mEq/l, after which the value can be checked monthly during oral Mg or diet therapy. A serum potassium level of >4 mEq/l illustrates effective Mg therapy; however, the value should not go above 5 mEq/l. The optimal range of serum potassium is 3.7–5.2 mEq/l.[111]

Unlike serum potassium, serum Mg does not necessarily reflect the whole-body status of Mg because the normal range used by many clinical laboratories for this measurement does not account for a chronic latent Mg deficit chronic latent magnesium deficit (CLMD).[4] Research recommends using 0.85 mmol/l, (which translates to 1.70 mEq/l or 2.07 mg/dl[112]) as the lower range of normal when assessing a patient's Mg sufficiency using serum Mg. Serum Mg responds to dietary changes, including supplementation, in months rather than weeks or days, whereas urinary Mg (24-hr) responds to a change in Mg intake within days.[113]

5. Assess your patient's magnesium status

Even if serum Mg is within the normal range, a patient may have low Mg stores or CLMD,[112] especially if Mg intake has been chronically low as for most individuals on a modern processed food diet. If serum Mg results are inconclusive, resources are available to further assess Mg status. For example, the ExaTest (www.Exatest.com) utilizes the patient's buccal cells. In addition, results from the Mg Status Questionnaire can prove helpful.[114] However, there is no reliable biological marker for overall Mg status. Nevertheless, physicians can safely opt to implement oral Mg therapy for their patients at an appropriate dose for 4–6 months. If the patient's high blood pressure is normalized, low HDL cholesterol increases, high LDL cholesterol decreases, and/or sodium excretion increases, it can be deduced that the patient had a baseline Mg deficit.[115]

6. Replenish your patient's potassium and magnesium

Methods for replenishing patients' potassium and Mg include making changes to their diet, using salt substitutes, adding a supplement, or any combination of all three. Patients can increase both Mg and potassium by adding more nuts, seeds, whole grains, legumes, fruits, and vegetables to their diet. Espresso coffee (decaffeinated or regular) can also be high in Mg and potassium. Patients can maximize the existing level of Mg in their diet by lowering the amounts of saturated fat, sugar, and refined carbohydrates and keeping their vitamin D and calcium in balance with Mg intake. They can also decrease their need for potassium by lowering their dietary sodium. These recommendations are contained in the following diets (DASH,[104] Ornish,[106] and Mediterranean Diet).[109] A program to make these changes is detailed in Chapter 11 of *The Magnesium Factor* by Seelig and Rosanoff[114] or any of the DASH books by Heller.[104]

If dietary changes are unrealistic for a patient or do not provide the desired result, physicians can add salt supplements to a patient's diet. If the dietary assessment or Mg questionnaire result shows a risk of low Mg status, or serum Mg is below 0.85 mmol/L, a Mg-containing salt (e.g., Cardia Salt by Nutrition 21, available on Amazon.com) in place of usual salt is recommended. Patients displaying a low risk for Mg deficiency who still experience hypertension may benefit from potassium salt substitutes with the goal of 4700 mg potassium/day from all sources. LiteSalt (from Morton Salt) contains half potassium and half sodium chloride and is a good option for patients who enjoy cooking, as it lends itself well to use in daily meals. This product contains about 340 mg potassium per 1/4 teaspoon. If a patient does not tend to cook his or her own meals, products such as Morton Salt Substitute or NoSalt could be considered. These products contain potassium chloride without sodium. (Of note, if the patient's Mg is low, products with just potassium will not be able to normalize high blood pressure.) NoSalt and Morton Salt Substitute contain approximately 680 mg potassium per 1/4 teaspoon.

Oral Mg supplements of about 600 mg elemental Mg/day for hypertensive patients who are treatment naïve or 350 mg elemental Mg/day for hypertensive patients taking anti-hypertensive medications should be adequate to normalize blood pressure or at least decrease it in 3–6 months.[12] If potassium supplements are deemed necessary, doses between 1780 and 7800 mg elemental potassium/day have been found both safe and effective in lowering high blood pressure.[80] It should be noted that caution should be used in chronic kidney disease patients.

For patients with kidney disease, physicians must proceed with caution when prescribing any pills or salt supplements containing substantial amounts of potassium or Mg by monitoring patients' serum Mg and/or potassium closely.

7. Gradually start to withdraw hypertension medication(s)

A few months after the patient initiates oral supplementation, a new diet, and/or salt substitute supplements, the physician can gradually begin withdrawing a patient's anti-hypertensive medications if blood pressure is decreasing. This taper should occur slowly by decreasing the patient's dose every 1–4 weeks while monitoring the patient's blood pressure.

8. If necessary, add traditional oral magnesium supplements to your patient's regimen

If the above salt substitute supplements do not fully normalize the patient's blood pressure or allow the patient to discontinue anti-hypertensive medications, the addition of Mg and/or potassium supplements should be initiated. In addition to the aforementioned dietary changes, 700 mg Mg/day can be added and then gradually titrated up to 1200 mg/day, giving each dose several weeks to work. (For patients taking anti-hypertensive medications, 240–500 mg elemental Mg/day should be adequate.) When Mg appears adequate, but hypertension is still evident, potassium repletion may begin. Potassium supplements can begin at 2600 mg/day and then be titrated up to 3600 (or higher, up to 7800 mg/day),[80] giving each dose at least 4–6 weeks to take effect. Caution is advised in chronic kidney disease patients. If a patient has had hypertension for an extended period of time, his or her blood pressure may not entirely normalize even as Mg and potassium status are brought into adequacy. Nonetheless, the risk factor for heart disease is the underlying Mg and/or potassium deficiency versus the hypertension itself. As such, patients can still reduce their risk of stroke and heart disease with adequate Mg/potassium status despite continued hypertension. The key to treatment success is to make gradual, rather than sudden, changes in the patient's nutritional status, as this allows the patient's body to normalize its blood pressure as it is slowly weaned from anti-hypertensive medications.

People with low serum Mg have shown a gradual decrease in serum Mg at 2–6 weeks of oral Mg therapy before the serum Mg increases into the normal range.[54] Other studies show blood pressure to remain stable during this 2- to 6-week period of Mg adjustment before decreasing significantly by 3 months.[39,56] In general, an oral daily dose of 200 mg Mg for 1 month has been shown to significantly raise serum Mg, but Mg doses above 300 mg/day for at least 2 months are necessary to achieve maximal/optimal serum Mg levels.[12] The latest and most comprehensive meta-analysis of Mg for blood pressure studies showed that a median oral Mg dose of 368 mg/day for a median of 3 months both raised serum Mg levels by an average of 0.05 mmol/L and significantly decreased both systolic and diastolic blood pressure.[12] However, this and other meta-analyses combined subjects who were either normotensive or hypertensive at baseline, were taking anti-hypertensive medications, or were treatment naïve. A close look at such studies has shown that oral Mg doses in treatment-naïve subjects need to be at least 600 mg Mg/day to show a significant decrease in a high blood pressure (Table 7.1), while lower doses, in the range of 240–350 mg/day, appear adequate in hypertensive subjects taking anti-hypertensive medications.[60] Some patients show a large blood pressure response to oral Mg therapy, whereas others show moderate or no blood pressure response. In general, those with a higher baseline blood pressure usually show the largest decrease in blood pressure with oral Mg therapy.[40,43,116] Attention should be paid to the following:

- the Mg dose so that it is appropriate for the anti-hypertensive medication usage (if any),
- the time of duration for oral Mg therapy (expecting at least a possible 3-month period to see lower blood pressure measurements and/or a rise in serum Mg), as well as
- the general health of the patient.

If oral Mg therapy successfully lowers blood pressure to <140/<90 without anti-hypertensive medications, the oral Mg supplement dose can be lowered to about 150–350 mg/day, depending on the patient's health status, diet, and use or non-use of transdermal Mg. A list of Mg deficiency symptoms is available online (http://www.magnesiumeducation.com/mg-deficiencies).

9. Consider injections for patients who do not adequately respond to oral therapy for hypertension

If a patient does not respond to more modest hypertension therapy (e.g., removal of potassium- and Mg-wasting medications, alteration of diet, use of salt substitutes that include Mg, and/or use of a transdermal Mg supplement), or to a round of oral Mg and/or potassium therapy of an appropriately high dose and 3- to 6-month duration, *and* serum potassium remains <4 mEq/l, Mg, then intramuscular injections may be considered. Mg sulfate serves as the more common choice for this purpose.

Patients with chronic hypomagnesemia receive intravenous or intramuscular Mg weekly. Guidelines for this treatment are discussed in Seelig and Rosanoff.[117]

Questions and answers

Is a high potassium intake dangerous?

When potassium is given intravenously in a hospital, too much potassium infused too fast can cause arrhythmias. In addition, potassium supplements can prove dangerous for patients with kidney disease and can lead to stomach ulcers. Nonetheless, potassium supplementation is generally safe when given orally to a patient with normal kidney function. Oral potassium doses of 1170–7800 mg/day have been shown to be both safe and effective in several studies.[80,118] Even long-term high potassium dietary intake is not associated with chronic problems in patients with healthy kidney function. A dietary intake of 3500 mg potassium/day is beneficial to health[118,119] but Mg status needs to be adequate for potassium to be optimally utilized by the body.

Is a low potassium intake dangerous?

In adults with healthy renal function, the benefits of adequate potassium intake far outweigh the low risk of hyperkalemia associated with medically monitored potassium supplementation. Low potassium status and/or intake is associated with higher risks for stroke, heart disease, and high bone turnover as well as muscle weakness, glucose intolerance, increased salt sensitiv3ity, hypertension, and/or increased risk of kidney stones.[118,120] When assessing your patients, remember that over 90% of the U.S. population (and every age/gender group) is consuming less than the adequate intake for potassium every day, while over 97% of every age group consumes above the adequate intake for sodium each and every day.[74]

Is a high magnesium intake dangerous?

Intravenous Mg is increasingly employed in clinical settings without harm. High-dose oral Mg can have a laxative effect in some people. If more Mg is absorbed than the body needs, normal kidneys rapidly pass any excess in the urine. Oral Mg supplements are very safe for patients with healthy kidney function. Hypermagnesemia can occur, however. Caution should be used in patients who have impaired kidney function.

Is a low magnesium intake dangerous?

Without enough Mg, many serious disorders can develop in the heart, arteries, and other tissues as well. Inflammation parameters[121] have been associated with low Mg intake/status, as have metabolic syndrome,[122] type 2 diabetes,[123] increased incidence of bone fractures,[124] migraines,[125] depression,[126-128] and other issues. See Seelig and Rosanoff[114] for a list of Mg deficit symptoms.

In summary

Most essential hypertension is a result of low Mg and/or potassium intake coupled with very high intakes of sodium. As such, it is the underlying deficiency in Mg (and/or potassium) that is associated with hypertension, rather than hypertension alone, that increases the risk for cardiovascular disease in individuals. Correcting high blood pressure without correcting Mg deficiency (if it exists) could fail to prevent cardiovascular disease and could worsen the individual's health, due to medication side effects or the high stress resulting from an inability to make lifestyle changes.

Some patients with normal blood pressure may be getting adequate amounts of Mg and need only to prevent the onset of high blood pressure by ensuring proper balanced micronutrition of Mg, potassium, sodium, and calcium. However, other patients with normal blood pressure can have sub-optimal or deficient Mg status. It should not be assumed that everyone with hypertension has an Mg deficit nor that everyone with normal blood pressure has adequate Mg status. For this reason, physician knowledge of the micronutrients Mg, calcium, potassium, and sodium is vital to achieving effective, safe treatment and preventing essential hypertension and its associated health risks.

References

1. Centers for Disease Control and Prevention. Vital signs: awareness and treatment of uncontrolled hypertension among adults – United States, 2003–2010. *MMWR Morb. Mortal. Wkly. Rep.* 2012;61:703–9.
2. World Health Organization. A global brief on hypertension: silent killer, global public health crisis (WHO reference number: WHO/DCO/WHD/2013.2 ed), 2013. http://www.who.int/cardiovascular_diseases/publications/global_brief_hypertension/en/. Accessed June 26, 2017.
3. American Heart Association. Statistical Fact Sheet 2013 Update: High Blood Pressure, 2013. https://www.heart.org/idc/groups/heart-public/@wcm/@sop/@smd/documents/downloadable/ucm_319587.pdf. Accessed June 26, 2017.
4. Rosanoff A, Weaver CM, Rude RK. Suboptimal magnesium status in the United States: are the health consequences underestimated? *Nutr. Rev.* 2012;70(3):153–64.
5. Rosanoff A. Changing crop magnesium concentrations: impact on human health. *Plant Soil.* 2013;368:139–53.
6. Lozano R, Naghavi M, Foreman K, et al. Global and regional mortality from 235 causes of death for 20 age groups in 1990 and 2010: a systematic analysis for the Global Burden of Disease Study 2010. *Lancet.* 2013;380(9859):2095–128.
7. Bayır A, Kara H, Ak A, Cander B, Kara F. Magnesium sulfate in emergency department patients with hypertension. *Biol. Trace. Elem. Res.* 2009;128(1):38–44.

8. Rosanoff A, Plesset MR. Oral magnesium supplements decrease high blood pressure (SBP> 155mmHg) in hypertensive subjects on anti-hypertensive medications: a targeted meta-analysis. *Magnes. Res.* 2013;26(3):93–9.
9. Dickinson HO, Nicolson DJ, Campbell F, et al. Magnesium supplementation for the management of essential hypertension in adults. *Cochrane Database Syst. Rev.* 2006;3:CD004640.
10. Jee SH, Miller ER, 3rd, Guallar E, Singh VK, Appel LJ, Klag MJ. The effect of magnesium supplementation on blood pressure: a meta-analysis of randomized clinical trials. *Am. J. Hypertens.* 2002;15(8):691–6.
11. Kass L, Weekes J, Carpenter L. Effect of magnesium supplementation on blood pressure: a meta-analysis. *Eur. J. Clin. Nutr.* 2012;66(4):411–8.
12. Zhang X, Li Y, Del Gobbo LC, et al. Effects of magnesium supplementation on blood pressure: a meta-analysis of randomized double-blind placebo-controlled trials. *Hypertension.* 2016;68(2):324–33.
13. Borrello G, Mastroroberto P, Curcio F, Chello M, Zofrea S, Mazza ML. The effects of magnesium oxide on mild essential hypertension and quality of life. *Curr. Therapeutic. Res.* 1996;57(10):767–74.
14. Nowson CA, Morgan TO. Magnesium supplementation in mild hypertensive patients on a moderately low sodium diet. *Clin. Exp. Pharmacol. Physiol.* 1989;16(4):299–302.
15. Ferrara LA, Iannuzzi R, Castaldo A, Iannuzzi A, Dello Russo A, Mancini M. Long-term magnesium supplementation in essential hypertension. *Cardiology.* 1992;81(1):25–33.
16. Lind L, Lithell H, Pollare T, Ljunghall S. Blood pressure response during long-term treatment with magnesium is dependent on magnesium status. A double-blind, placebo-controlled study in essential hypertension and in subjects with high-normal blood pressure. *Am. J. Hypertens.* 1991;4(8):674–9.
17. de Valk HW, Verkaaik R, van Rijn HJ, Geerdink RA, Struyvenberg A. Oral magnesium supplementation in insulin-requiring type 2 diabetic patients. *Diabet. Med.* 1998;15(6):503–7.
18. Plum-Wirell M, Stegmayr B, Wester P. Nutritional magnesium supplementation does not change blood pressure nor serum or muscle potassium and magnesium in untreated hypertension. A double-blind crossover study. *Magnes. Res.* 1994;7(3–4):277–83.
19. Wirell MM, Wester PO, Stegmayr BG. Nutritional dose of magnesium given to short-term thiazide treated hypertensive patients does not alter the blood pressure or the magnesium and potassium in muscle – a double blind crossover study. *Magnes. Bull.* 1993;15(2):50–4.
20. Cappuccio FP, Markandu ND, Beynon GW, Shore AC, Sampson B, MacGregor GA. Lack of effect of oral magnesium on high blood pressure: a double blind study. *Br. Med. J. (Clin. Res. Ed.).* 1985;291(6490):235–8.
21. Reyes AJ, Leary WP, Acosta-Barrios TN, Davis WH. Magnesium supplementation in hypertension treated with hydrochlorothiazide. *Curr. Ther. Res.* 1984;36(2):332–40.
22. Olhaberry J, Reyes AJ, Acosta-Barrios TN, Leary WP, Queiruga G. Pilot evaluation of the putative antihypertensive effect of magnesium. *Magnes. Bull.* 1987;9:181–4.
23. Purvis JR, Cummings DM, Landsman P, et al. Effect of oral magnesium supplementation on selected cardiovascular risk factors in non-insulin-dependent diabetics. *Arch. Fam. Med.* 1994;3(6):503–8.

24. Witteman JC, Grobbee DE, Derkx FH, Bouillon R, de Bruijn AM, Hofman A. Reduction of blood pressure with oral magnesium supplementation in women with mild to moderate hypertension. *Am. J. Clin. Nutr.* 1994;60(1):129–35.

25. Patki PS, Singh J, Gokhale SV, Bulakh PM, Shrotri DS, Patwardhan B. Efficacy of potassium and magnesium in essential hypertension: a double-blind, placebo controlled, crossover study. *BMJ.* 1990;301(6751):521–3.

26. Walker AF, Marakis G, Morris AP, Robinson PA. Promising hypotensive effect of hawthorn extract: a randomized double-blind pilot study of mild, essential hypertension. *Phytother. Res.* 2002;16(1):48–54.

27. Haga H. Effects of dietary magnesium supplementation on diurnal variations of blood pressure and plasma Na+, K(+)-ATPase activity in essential hypertension. *Jpn. Heart. J.* 1992;33(6):785–800.

28. Motoyama T, Sano H, Fukuzaki H. Oral magnesium supplementation in patients with essential hypertension. *Hypertension.* 1989;13(3):227–32.

29. Sanjuliani AF, de Abreu Fagundes VG, Francischetti EA. Effects of magnesium on blood pressure and intracellular ion levels of Brazilian hypertensive patients. *Int. J. Cardiol.* 1996;56(2):177–83.

30. Zemel PC, Zemel MB, Urberg M, Douglas FL, Geiser R, Sowers JR. Metabolic and hemodynamic effects of magnesium supplementation in patients with essential hypertension. *Am. J. Clin. Nutr.* 1990;51(4):665–9.

31. Widman L, Wester PO, Stegmayr BK, Wirell M. The dose-dependent reduction in blood pressure through administration of magnesium A double blind placebo controlled cross-over study. *Am. J. Hypertens.* 1993;6(1):41–5.

32. Shafique M, Misbah ul A, Ashraf M. Role of magnesium in the management of hypertension. *J. Pak. Med. Assoc.* 1993;43(4):77–8.

33. Sebekova K, Revusova V, Polakovicova D, Drahosova J, Zverkova D, Dzurik R. Anti-hypertensive treatment with magnesium-aspartate-dichloride and its influence on peripheral serotonin metabolism in man: a subacute study. *Cor Vasa.* 1992;34(5–6):390–401.

34. Michón P. [Level of total and ionized magnesium fraction based on biochemical analysis of blood and hair and effect of supplemented magnesium (Slow Mag B6) on selected parameters in hypertension of patients treated with various groups of drugs]. *Ann. Acad. Med. Stetin.* 2002;48:85–97.

35. Wirell MP, Wester PO, Stegmayr BG. Nutritional dose of magnesium in hypertensive patients on beta blockers lowers systolic blood pressure: a double-blind, cross-over study. *J. Intern. Med.* 1994;236(2):189–95.

36. Dyckner T, Wester PO. Effect of magnesium on blood pressure. *Br. Med. J. (Clin. Res. Ed.).* 1983;286(6381):1847–9.

37. Rodriguez-Moran M, Guerrero-Romero F. Oral magnesium supplementation improves the metabolic profile of metabolically obese, normal-weight individuals: a randomized double-blind placebo-controlled trial. *Arch. Med. Res.* 2014;45(5):388–93.

38. Paolisso G, Di Maro G, Cozzolino D, et al. Chronic magnesium administration enhances oxidative glucose metabolism in thiazide treated hypertensive patients. *Am. J. Hypertens.* 1992;5(10):681–6.

39. Guerrero-Romero F, Rodriguez-Moran M. The effect of lowering blood pressure by magnesium supplementation in diabetic hypertensive adults with low serum magnesium levels: a randomized, double-blind, placebo-controlled clinical trial. *J. Hum. Hypertens.* 2009;23(4):245–51.

40. Kawano Y, Matsuoka H, Takishita S, Omae T. Effects of magnesium supplementation in hypertensive patients: assessment by office, home, and ambulatory blood pressures. *Hypertension.* 1998;32(2):260–5.
41. Saito K, Hattori K, Omatsu T, Hirouchi H, Sano H, Fukuzaki H. Effects of oral magnesium on blood pressure and red cell sodium transport in patients receiving long-term thiazide diuretics for hypertension. *Am. J. Hypertens.* 1988;1(3 Pt 3):71S–4S.
42. Doyle L, Flynn A, Cashman K. The effect of magnesium supplementation on biochemical markers of bone metabolism or blood pressure in healthy young adult females. *Eur. J. Clin. Nutr.* 1999;53(4):255–61.
43. Lee S, Park HK, Son SP, Lee CW, Kim IJ, Kim HJ. Effects of oral magnesium supplementation on insulin sensitivity and blood pressure in normo-magnesemic nondiabetic overweight Korean adults. *Nutr. Metab. Cardiovasc. Dis.* 2009;19(11):781–8.
44. Henderson DG, Schierup J, Schodt T. Effect of magnesium supplementation on blood pressure and electrolyte concentrations in hypertensive patients receiving long term diuretic treatment. *Br. Med. J. (Clin. Res. Ed.)* 1986;293(6548):664–5.
45. Guerrero-Romero F, Tamez-Perez HE, Gonzalez-Gonzalez G, et al. Oral magnesium supplementation improves insulin sensitivity in non-diabetic subjects with insulin resistance. A double-blind placebo-controlled randomized trial. *Diabetes Metab.* 2004;30(3):253–8.
46. Sacks FM, Willett WC, Smith A, Brown LE, Rosner B, Moore TJ. Effect on blood pressure of potassium, calcium, and magnesium in women with low habitual intake. *Hypertension.* 1998;31(1):131–8.
47. TOHP Study Group. The effects of nonpharmacologic interventions on blood pressure of persons with high normal levels. Results of the Trials of Hypertension Prevention, Phase I. *JAMA.* 1992;267(9):1213–20.
48. Mooren FC, Kruger K, Volker K, Golf SW, Wadephul M, Kraus A. Oral magnesium supplementation reduces insulin resistance in non-diabetic subjects – a double-blind, placebo-controlled, randomized trial. *Diabetes Obes. Metab.* 2011;13:281–4.
49. Sibai BM, Villar MA, Bray E. Magnesium supplementation during pregnancy: a double-blind randomized controlled clinical trial. *Am. J. Obstet. Gynecol.* 1989;161(1):115–9.
50. Sacks FM, Brown LE, Appel L, Borhani NO, Evans D, Whelton P. Combinations of potassium, calcium, and magnesium supplements in hypertension. *Hypertension.* 1995;26(6 Pt 1):950–6.
51. Simental-Mendia LE, Rodriguez-Moran M, Guerrero-Romero F. Oral magnesium supplementation decreases C-reactive protein levels in subjects with prediabetes and hypomagnesemia: a clinical randomized double-blind placebo-controlled trial. *Arch. Med. Res.* 2014;45(4):325–30.
52. Cosaro E, Bonafini S, Montagnana M, et al. Effects of magnesium supplements on blood pressure, endothelial function and metabolic parameters in healthy young men with a family history of metabolic syndrome. *Nutr. Metab. Cardiovasc. Dis.* 2014;24(11):1213–20.
53. Itoh K, Kawasaka T, Nakamura M. The effects of high oral magnesium supplementation on blood pressure, serum lipids and related variables in apparently healthy Japanese subjects. *Br. J. Nutr.* 1997;78(5):737–50.

54. Rodriguez-Moran M, Guerrero-Romero F. Oral magnesium supplementation improves insulin sensitivity and metabolic control in type 2 diabetic subjects: a randomized double-blind controlled trial. *Diabetes Care.* 2003;26(4):1147–52.

55. Rodriguez-Hernandez H, Cervantes-Huerta M, Rodriguez-Moran M, Guerrero-Romero F. Oral magnesium supplementation decreases alanine aminotransferase levels in obese women. *Magnes. Res.* 2010;23(2):90–6.

56. Daly NM, Allen KGD, Harris M. Magnesium supplementation and blood pressure in borderline hypertensive subjects: a double blind study. *Magnes. Bull.* 1990;12(4):149–54.

57. Kisters K, Spieker C, Tepel M, Zidek W. New data about the effects of oral physiological magnesium supplementation on several cardiovascular risk factors (lipids and blood pressure). *Magnes. Res.* 1993;6(4):355–60.

58. Wary C, Brillault-Salvat C, Bloch G, et al. Effect of chronic magnesium supplementation on magnesium distribution in healthy volunteers evaluated by 31P-NMRS and ion selective electrodes. *Br. J. Clin. Pharmacol.* 1999;48(5):655–62.

59. Guerrero-Romero F, Rodriguez-Moran M. Magnesium improves the beta-cell function to compensate variation of insulin sensitivity: double-blind, randomized clinical trial. *Eur. J. Clin. Invest.* 2011;41(4):405–10.

60. Rosanoff A. Magnesium supplements may enhance the effect of antihypertensive medications in stage 1 hypertensive subjects. *Magnes. Res.* 2010;23(1):27–40.

61. Di Bianco R Captopril in the treatment of congestive heart failure. *Herz.* 1987;12:27–37.

62. Dietz R, Osterziel K. Effects of angiotensin-converting enzyme inhibitors in heart failure. *Zeitschrift fur Kardiologie.* 1988;77:89–93.

63. Leary WP. Renal excretory actions of antihypertensive agents: effects of rilmenidine. *Am. J. Med.* 1989;87(3):S63–6.

64. Reyes AJ. Mechanisms and extent of the decrease in magnesiuresis induced by antikaliuretic diuretics in man. *Magnesium in Health and Disease.* London: John Libbey; 1989:415–22.

65. Stevenson R, Keywood C, Amadi A, Davies J, Patterson D. Angiotensin converting enzyme inhibitors and magnesium conservation in patients with congestive cardiac failure. *Heart.* 1991;66(1):19–21.

66. Oladapo O, Falase A. Congestive heart failure and ventricular arrhythmias in relation to serum magnesium. *Afr. J. Med. Med. Sci.* 2000;29(3–4):265–8.

67. Haenni A, Berglund L, Reneland R, Anderssson P-E, Lind L, Lithell H. The alterations in insulin sensitivity during angiotensin converting enzyme inhibitor treatment are related to changes in the calcium/magnesium balance. *Am. J. Hypertens.* 1997;10(2):145–51.

68. Landmark K, Urdal P, Landmark K. Serum magnesium and potassium in acute myocardial infarction: relationship to existing β-blockade and infarct size. *Angiology.* 1993;44(5):347–52.

69. O'Keeffe S, Grimes H, Finn J, McMurrough P, Daly K. Effect of captopril therapy on lymphocyte potassium and magnesium concentrations in patients with congestive heart failure. *Cardiology.* 1992;80(2):100–5.

70. Barbagallo M, Dominguez LJ, Resnick LM. Protective effects of captopril against ischemic stress: role of cellular Mg. *Hypertension.* 1999;34(4 Pt 2):958–63.

71. Kuller L, Farrier N, Caggiula A, Borhani N, Dunkle S. Relationship of diuretic therapy and serum magnesium levels among participants in the Multiple Risk Factor Intervention Trial. *Am. J. Epidemiol.* 1985;122(6):1045–59.
72. Turlapaty PD, Altura BM. Magnesium deficiency produces spasms of coronary arteries: relationship to etiology of sudden death ischemic heart disease. *Science.* 1980;208(4440):198–200.
73. Resnick L. The cellular ionic basis of hypertension and allied clinical conditions. *Prog. Cardiovasc. Dis.* 1999;42(1):1–22.
74. Moshfegh A, Goldman J, Cleveland L. What We Eat in America, NHANES 2001–2002: Usual Nutrient Intakes from Food Compared to Dietary Reference Intakes, 2005, pp. 34 and 35. http://www.ars.usda.gov/SP2UserFiles/Place/12355000/pdf/0102/usualintaketables2001-02.pdf. Accessed June 5, 2017.
75. Conlin PR. The dietary approaches to stop hypertension (DASH) clinical trial: implications for lifestyle modifications in the treatment of hypertensive patients. *Cardiol. Rev.* 1998;7(5):284–8.
76. Kwan MW, Wong MC, Wang HH, et al. Compliance with the Dietary Approaches to Stop Hypertension (DASH) diet: a systematic review. *PLoS One.* 2013;8(10):e78412.
77. Harrington JM, Fitzgerald AP, Kearney PM, et al. DASH diet score and distribution of blood pressure in middle-aged men and women. *Am. J. Hypertens.* 2013;26(11):1311–20.
78. Addison WL. The use of sodium chloride, potassium chloride, sodium bromide, and potassium bromide in cases of arterial hypertension which are amenable to potassium chloride. *Can. Med. Assoc. J.* 1928;18 (3):281–5.
79. Priddle WW. Observations on the management of hypertension. *Can. Med. Assoc. J.* 1931;25(1):5–8.
80. Poorolajal J, Zeraati F, Soltanian AR, Sheikh V, Hooshmand E, Maleki A. Oral potassium supplementation for management of essential hypertension: a meta-analysis of randomized controlled trials. *PLoS One.* 2017;12(4):e0174967.
81. Seelig MS, Rosanoff A. High Blood Pressure, Salt and Magnesium. *The Magnesium Factor.* New York: Avery Penguin Group; 2003:53–8, 316–7.
82. Shils ME. Experimental human magnesium depletion. *Medicine (Baltimore).* 1969;48(1):61–85.
83. Mitka M. DASH dietary plan could benefit many, but few hypertensive patients follow it. *JAMA.* 2007;298(2):164–65.
84. Zhang A, Cheng TP, Altura BM. Magnesium regulates intracellular free ionized calcium concentration and cell geometry in vascular smooth muscle cells. *Biochim. Biophys. Acta.* 1992;1134(1):25–9.
85. Altura B, Zhang A, Altura B. Magnesium, hypertensive vascular diseases, atherogenesis, subcellular compartmentation of Ca2+ and Mg2+ and vascular contractility. *Miner. Electrolyte. Metab.* 1993;19(4–5):323–36.
86. Cox RH, Lozinskaya I, Dietz NJ. Calcium exerts a larger regulatory effect on potassium+ channels in small mesenteric artery mycoytes from spontaneously hypertensive rats compared to Wistar-Kyoto rats. *Am. J. Hypertens.* 2003;16(1):21–7.
87. Sela S, Shurtz-Swirski R, Farah R, et al. A link between polymorphonuclear leukocyte intracellular calcium, plasma insulin, and essential hypertension. *Am. J. Hypertens.* 2002;15(4 Pt 1):291–5.

88. Haenni A, Fugmann A, Lind L, Lithell H. Systolic blood pressure alterations during hyperinsulinemia are related to changes in ionized calcium status. *Am. J. Hypertens.* 2001;14(11):1106–11.

89. Camilletti A, Moretti N, Giacchetti G, et al. Decreased nitric oxide levels and increased calcium content in platelets of hypertensive patients. *Am. J. Hypertens.* 2001;14(4):382–6.

90. Meyer-Lehnert H, Bäcker A, Kramer HJ. Inhibitors of Na-K-ATPase in human urine: effects of ouabain-like factors and of vanadium-diascorbate on calcium mobilization in rat vascular smooth muscle cells. *Am. J. Hypertens.* 2000;13(4):364–9.

91. Shimosawa T, Takano K, Ando K, Fujita T. Magnesium inhibits norepinephrine release by blocking N-type calcium channels at peripheral sympathetic nerve endings. *Hypertension.* 2004;44(6):897–902.

92. Kisters K, Wessels F, Küper H, et al. Increased calcium and decreased magnesium concentrations and an increased calcium/magnesium ratio in spontaneously hypertensive rats versus Wistar-Kyoto rats: relation to arteriosclerosis. *Am. J. Hypertens.* 2004;17(1):59–62.

93. Seelig MS. The requirement of magnesium by the normal adult Summary and analysis of published data. *Am. J. Clin. Nutr.* 1964;14(6):342–90.

94. Alderman MH, Lamport B. Moderate sodium restriction. Do the benefits justify the hazards? *Am. J. Hypertens.* 1990;3(6 Pt 1):499–504.

95. Graudal NA, Galloe AM, Garred P. Effects of sodium restriction on blood pressure, renin, aldosterone, catecholamines, cholesterols, and triglyceride: a meta-analysis. *JAMA.* 1998;279(17):1383–91.

96. Esslinger KA, Jones PJ. Dietary sodium intake and mortality. *Nutr. Rev.* 1998;56(10):311–3.

97. Alderman MH, Madhavan S, Cohen H, Sealey JE, Laragh JH. Low urinary sodium is associated with greater risk of myocardial infarction among treated hypertensive men. *Hypertension.* 1995;25(6):1144–52.

98. McCarron DA. Role of adequate dietary calcium intake in the prevention and management of salt-sensitive hypertension. *Am. J. Clin. Nutr.* 1997;65(2 Suppl):712S–6S.

99. Hurley SW, Johnson AK. The biopsychology of salt hunger and sodium deficiency. *Pflugers. Arch.* 2015;467(3):445–56.

100. Dineen R, Thompson CJ, Sherlock M. Hyponatraemia–presentations and management. *Clin. Med.* 2017;17(3):263–9.

101. Rosanoff A, Clemens R. Food, medicine & health managing magnesium in a sodium-dominant era. *Food Technol.* 2010;64(6):21.

102. Kass L, Sullivan KR. Low dietary magnesium intake and hypertension. *World J. Cardiovas. Dis.* 2016;6(12):447.

103. US Department of Agriculture. What We Eat In America, NHANES 2013–14, Individuals 2 years and over (excluding breast-fed children), day 1, 2016. http://www.ars.usda.gov/nea/bhnrc/fsrg. Accessed October 13, 2016.

104. Heller M. What is the DASH Diet?, 2016. http://dashdiet.org/what_is_the_dash_diet.asp Accessed June 22, 2017.

105. Lin P-H, Aickin M, Champagne C, et al. Food group sources of nutrients in the dietary patterns of the DASH-Sodium trial. *J. Am. Diet. Assoc.* 2003;103(4):488–96.

106. Ornish D. *Dr. Dean Ornish's Program for Reversing Heart Disease: The Only System Scientifically Proven to Reverse Heart Disease Without Drugs or Surgery.* New York: Ivy Books; 1996.
107. Ornish D, Scherwitz LW, Billings JH, et al. Intensive lifestyle changes for reversal of coronary heart disease. *JAMA.* 1998;280(23):2001–7.
108. Seelig MS. Consequences of magnesium deficiency on the enhancement of stress reactions; preventive and therapeutic implications (a review). *J. Am. Coll. Nutr.* 1994;13(5):429–46.
109. Romaguera D, Norat T, Mouw T, et al. Adherence to the Mediterranean diet is associated with lower abdominal adiposity in European men and women. *J. Nutr.* 2009;139(9):1728–37.
110. Kass L, Rosanoff A, Tanner A, Sullivan K, McAuley W, Plesset M. Effect of transdermal magnesium cream on serum and urinary magnesium levels in humans: a pilot study. *PLoS One.* 2017;12(4):e0174817.
111. US National Library of Medicine. MedlinePlus Medical Encyclopedia: Comprehensive Metabolic panel, 2017. https://medlineplus.gov/ency/article/003468.htm. Accessed July 5, 2017.
112. Elin RJ. Re-evaluation of the concept of chronic, latent, magnesium deficiency. *Magnes. Res.* 2011;24(4):225–7.
113. Nielsen FH, Johnson L. Data from controlled metabolic ward studies provide guidance for the determination of status indicators and dietary requirements for magnesium. *Biol. Trace. Elem. Res.* 2017;177(1):43–52.
114. Seelig MS, Rosanoff A. *The Magnesium Factor.* New York: Avery Penguin Group; 2003.
115. Lundberg GD. Magnesium Deficiency: The Real Emperor of All Maladies?, 2015. http://www.medscape.com/viewarticle/844214. Accessed July 5, 2017.
116. Rosanoff A, Plesset M. Successful treatment of hypertension with Mg—a targeted approach. In: Guerrero-Romero F, ed. *XIIXIII International Magnesium Symposium; Merida, Yucutan, Mexico; October 16–19,* 2012. Paris, France: International Society for the Development of Research on Magnesium; 2012.
117. Seelig MS, Rosanoff A. Appendix F: Guidelines for Magnesium Injections. *The Magnesium Factor.* New York: Avery Penguin Group; 2003:280–1.
118. Institute of Medicine, Water. *Dietary Reference Intakes for Water, Potassium, Sodium, Chloride, and Sulfate.* Washington, DC: National Academies Press; 2005.
119. Aburto NJ, Hanson S, Gutierrez H, Hooper L, Elliott P, Cappuccio FP. Effect of increased potassium intake on cardiovascular risk factors and disease: systematic review and meta-analyses. *BMJ.* 2013;346:f1378.
120. Adebamowo SN, Spiegelman D, Flint AJ, Willett WC, Rexrode KM. Intakes of magnesium, potassium, and calcium and the risk of stroke among men. *Int. J. Stroke.* 2015;10(7):1093–100.
121. Simental-Mendia LE, Sahebkar A, Rodriguez-Moran M, Zambrano-Galvan G, Guerrero-Romero F. Effect of magnesium supplementation on plasma C-reactive protein concentrations: a systematic review and meta-analysis of randomized controlled trials (published ahead of print May 25, 2017). *Curr. Pharm. Des.* doi:10.2174/1381612823666170525153605.
122. Guerrero-Romero F, Jaquez-Chairez FO, Rodriguez-Moran M. Magnesium in metabolic syndrome: a review based on randomized, double-blind clinical trials. *Magnes. Res.* 2016;29(4):146–53.

123. Larsson SC, Wolk A. Magnesium intake and risk of type 2 diabetes: a meta-analysis. *J. Intern. Med.* 2007;262(2):208–14.
124. Veronese N, Stubbs B, Solmi M, et al. Dietary magnesium intake and fracture risk: data from a large prospective study (published ahead of print June 20, 2017). *Br. J. Nutr.* doi:10.1017/S0007114517001350.
125. Chiu HY, Yeh TH, Huang YC, Chen PY. Effects of intravenous and oral magnesium on reducing migraine: a meta-analysis of randomized controlled trials. *Pain Physician.* 2016;19(1):E97–112.
126. Yary T, Aazami S, Soleimannejad K. Dietary intake of magnesium may modulate depression. *Biol. Trace. Elem. Res.* 2013;151(3):324–9.
127. Cheungpasitporn W, Thongprayoon C, Mao MA, et al. Hypomagnesaemia linked to depression: a systematic review and meta-analysis. *Intern. Med. J.* 2015;45(4):436–40.
128. Serefko A, Szopa A, Wlaz P, et al. Magnesium in depression. *Pharmacol. Rep.* 2013;65(3):547–54.

chapter eight

Magnesium therapy in stroke

Brian Silver

Contents

Introduction

There has been much interest in the application of magnesium treatment in the prevention and treatment of stroke. The study of magnesium as it applies to stroke has matured from observational studies to randomized controlled trials. The lessons learned from these studies have greatly enhanced the science behind magnesium treatment and stroke. The following review summarizes these studies and frames the current concept of magnesium as a treatment in stroke.

Putative mechanisms of the magnesium effect in stroke

The putative mechanism of magnesium effect on cerebrovascular disease in the brain is uncertain. Increased magnesium concentrations reduce the release of glutamate[1] and block N-methyl-D-aspartate receptors.[2] Other effects of magnesium include the potentiation of adenosine activity and the blocking of calcium entry into cells through the modulation of voltage-gated channels. In rabbit models, increased consumption of magnesium prolonged clotting time, decreased the concentration of total cholesterol, and decreased the severity of atherosclerosis in the aorta.[3] Very high magnesium diets may be hazardous based on a hypertensive rat study showing an increased risk of stroke mortality.[4]

Primary prevention

Large population-based studies have evaluated the association between magnesium intake and the occurrence of stroke. The Health Professionals Follow-Up Study, which began in 1986 and included 51,529 health professionals between the ages of 40 and 75, studied the relationship between magnesium intake and the risk of stroke over a follow-up period of 8 years.[5] Participants completed a 131-item food frequency questionnaire at study entry. During 323,394 person-years of follow-up, 328 participants suffered a stroke, including 210 ischemic, 70 hemorrhagic, and 48 unclassified strokes. Median magnesium intake ranged from 243 mg/dL in the lowest quintile to 452 mg/dL in the highest. The age-adjusted risk of stroke was 38% less in the highest quintile of magnesium consumption compared with the lowest. In a multivariate model, after adjusting for total energy intake, smoking, alcohol consumption, hypertension, hypercholesterolemia, parental history of myocardial infarction, profession, body mass index, and physical activity risk, there was a 30% reduction in the risk of stroke in the highest quintile of magnesium consumption compared with the lowest. Of note, the risk was strongly modified by a history of hypertension; that is, those without hypertension had no reduction in stroke risk with increasing magnesium consumption, while those with hypertension had a significant attenuation of risk with increasing magnesium consumption. In another study evaluating 26,556 Finnish male smokers aged 50–69, the highest quintile of magnesium consumption was associated with a 15% reduction in stroke compared with the lower quintile.[6] The effect was particularly prominent in men under 60 with the highest magnesium intake, in whom stroke risk was 24% lower compared with the lowest.

In women, by contrast, the findings on the relationship between magnesium consumption and stroke risk has been mixed. The Nurses' Health Study, which included 85,764 women aged 34–59, followed subjects for 1.16 million person-years of follow-up by 1994, during which time 690 new strokes occurred.[7] Of these, 386 were ischemic stroke, 129 were subarachnoid hemorrhage, 74 were intracerebral hemorrhage, and 101 were of undetermined type. A 61-item food questionnaire was administered at the beginning of the study in 1980. Median magnesium intake ranged from 211 mg/dL in the lowest quintile to 381 mg/dL in the highest quintile. No statistically significant relationship between quintile of magnesium consumption and risk of stroke was found in both adjusted and unadjusted models. Further, women who used magnesium supplements also did not have a reduction in ischemic stroke risk ($p = 0.28$). In the Women's Health Study, 39,786 women aged 39–89 who were followed for a median of 10 years had a food frequency questionnaire administered at baseline, including magnesium consumption.[8] Those in the highest quintile of magnesium consumption had a 13% lower risk of stroke compared with those in the lowest quintile. However, the risk of coronary heart disease in this cohort was not reduced.

A meta-analysis of 40 studies from nine countries, which included more than 1 million men and women and 67,261 cardiovascular events, compared outcomes based on magnesium consumption.[9] A progressive nonlinear decrease in stroke risk occurred as sodium consumption increased from 150 to 550 mg daily. The dose-response analysis showed a 7% decrease in stroke risk for each 100 mg/day increase in magnesium consumption.

Simply looking at environmental levels of magnesium rather than assessing consumption through food questionnaires may lead to varying conclusions regarding the relationship between magnesium and stroke. In the REGARDS study, which included 30,239 participants, there was no relationship between environmental magnesium levels and stroke risk.[10] However, a meta-analysis of magnesium content in the water supply did suggest a reduced risk of stroke mortality.[11]

Future studies of magnesium supplementation in certain populations (e.g., men with hypertension) would be of interest.

Acute treatment

The most active area of investigation into magnesium treatment has been acute stroke. Studies have focused on both ischemic stroke treatment and the prevention of vasospasm following aneurysmal subarachnoid hemorrhage. The first published large randomized trial of magnesium in acute ischemic stroke was IMAGES in 2004.[12] Based on the findings of benefit in animal models of acute stroke and promising results in a small pilot trial, investigators in 13 countries randomly allocated 2589 patients within 12 hours of the onset of acute ischemic stroke to 16 mMol of magnesium sulfate intravenously over 15 minutes followed by 65 mMol over 24 hours or placebo. A global outcome statistic at 90 days was the primary outcome measure. Median time to treatment was 7 hours. No statistically significant difference between treatment assignments was found, nor was there a difference in patients treated under 6 hours versus those treated later. Further, no differences were seen in those with cortical versus subcortical strokes, and those with ischemic stroke versus hemorrhagic stroke. No results regarding the interaction between magnesium (e.g., a neuroprotective effect pending definitive reperfusion) and thrombolytic therapy were reported in the trial. At the time the trial was conducted, endovascular therapy was not commonly performed, so no conclusions could be drawn with respect to the interaction between magnesium treatment and mechanical thrombectomy.

Approximately 10 years later, the FAST-MAG trial was reported and was the first large-scale study to use pre-hospital treatment as a means of earlier treatment within the time window of the stroke.[13] Treatment was initiated in one of 315 paramedic-staffed ambulances who then brought patients to one of 60 receiving hospitals sites in Los Angeles and Orange counties. Seventeen hundred patients with suspected stroke were randomly assigned to treatment with magnesium sulfate or placebo beginnings within 2 hours of symptom onset. Only 3.9% of patients had stroke mimics, while 73.3% had ischemic stroke, and 3.9% had intracerebral hemorrhage, indicating that the target population had been reached. The median time to start of magnesium sulfate from symptom onset was 45 minutes, by far the fastest time to treatment in any stroke trial. Despite the success of early treatment initiation, magnesium sulfate was no better than placebo at improving 90 day clinical outcomes. Approximately one-third of patients received thrombolytic therapy for acute ischemic stroke, but no treatment interaction with magnesium was found. Further, those treated in less than 60 minutes did not have a statistically significant benefit compared with those treated between 60 and 120 minutes. No analysis of patients receiving endovascular therapy was performed because such treatment was not proven until after the study was published.

The use of magnesium for the reversal of cerebral vasospasm has been tested in two randomized controlled trials: Magnesium and Acetylsalicylic acid in Subarachnoid Hemorrhage (MASH) [14] and MASH-2.[15] Delayed cerebral ischemia due to vasospasm occurs in approximately one-third of all patients with aneurysmal subarachnoid hemorrhage. Approximately 70% are left dead or disabled following the initial event. Based on animal studies showing reversal of vasospasm and reduction in infarct volume, human randomized trials were undertaken to evaluate the potential of magnesium in this disease state. MASH was conducted between 2000 and 2004 in multiple centers in the Netherlands; 283 patients were randomized to magnesium sulfate 64 mMol/L per day or placebo within 4 days of subarachnoid hemorrhage and continued until 14 days after occlusion of the aneurysm. After 3 months, delayed cerebral ischemia, the primary outcome measure, was reduced by 34%, though the result was not statistically significant. Death or significant disability, the secondary outcome measure, was reduced by 23%, again not statistically significant. On the strength of the findings, the investigators launched a larger study to definitely determine whether magnesium treatment improved clinical outcomes at 3 months. The second study, MASH-2, published in 2012, was conducted at multiple centers in the Netherlands, Scotland, and Chile between 2004 and 2011. Using the same protocol as the first study, 1204 patients were enrolled. At 90 days, the rate of poor outcome was 26.2% in the placebo group and 25.3% in the magnesium group, a result that was not statistically significant. The authors conducted a meta-analysis of this with six other smaller studies of magnesium in subarachnoid hemorrhage, totaling 2047 patients, and found no benefit of magnesium over placebo.

Secondary prevention and stroke recovery

At this time, no human studies of magnesium supplementation to reduce the chance of second stroke or to enhance stroke recovery have been published, nor have there been animal studies evaluating the potential effect of treatment during these time frames.

Conclusion and areas for future study

Though much has been learned about the effect of magnesium in the primary prevention of stroke and during its acute treatment, there are still areas of uncertainty. A randomized trial of magnesium supplementation for primary and secondary stroke prevention would be needed to definitively determine whether there are benefits. Preliminary data on the effects of magnesium supplementation during the period of stroke recovery would be needed to determine whether additional studies are warranted.

References

1. Lin JY, Chung SY, Lin MC, Cheng FC. Effects of magnesium sulfate on energy metabolites and glutamate in the cortex during focal cerebral ischemia and reperfusion in the gerbil monitored by a dual-probe microdialysis technique. *Life Sci* 2002;71:803–11.
2. Nowak L, Bregestovski P, Ascher P, Herbet A, Prochiantz A. Magnesium gates glutamate-activated channels in mouse central neurones. *Nature* 1984;307:462–5.
3. Renaud S, Ciavatti M, Thevenon C, Ripoll JP. Protective effects of dietary calcium and magnesium on platelet function and atherosclerosis in rabbits fed saturated fat. *Atherosclerosis* 1983;47:187–98.
4. Ganguli M, Tobian L, Sugimoto T. High magnesium diets increase blood pressure and enhance stroke mortality in hypertensive SHRsp rats. *Am J Hypertens* 1989;2:780–3.
5. Ascherio A, Rimm EB, Hernan MA, et al. Intake of potassium, magnesium, calcium, and fiber and risk of stroke among US men. *Circulation* 1998;98:1198–204.
6. Larsson SC, Virtanen MJ, Mars M, et al. Magnesium, calcium, potassium, and sodium intakes and risk of stroke in male smokers. *Arch Intern Med* 2008;168:459–65.
7. Iso H, Stampfer MJ, Manson JE, et al. Prospective study of calcium, potassium, and magnesium intake and risk of stroke in women. *Stroke* 1999;30:1772–9.
8. Song Y, Manson JE, Cook NR, Albert CM, Buring JE, Liu S. Dietary magnesium intake and risk of cardiovascular disease among women. *Am J Cardiol* 2005;96:1135–41.

9. Fang X, Wang K, Han D, et al. Dietary magnesium intake and the risk of cardiovascular disease, type 2 diabetes, and all-cause mortality: A dose-response meta-analysis of prospective cohort studies. *BMC Med* 2016;14:210.

10. Merrill PD, Ampah SB, He K, et al. Association between trace elements in the environment and stroke risk: The reasons for geographic and racial differences in stroke (REGARDS) study. *J Trace Elem Med Biol* 2017;42:45–9.

11. Yang CY. Calcium and magnesium in drinking water and risk of death from cerebrovascular disease. *Stroke* 1998;29:411–4.

12. Muir KW, Lees KR, Ford I, Davis S. Magnesium for acute stroke (Intravenous Magnesium Efficacy in Stroke trial): Randomised controlled trial. *Lancet* 2004;363:439–45.

13. Saver JL, Starkman S, Eckstein M, et al. Prehospital use of magnesium sulfate as neuroprotection in acute stroke. *N Engl J Med* 2015;372:528–36.

14. van den Bergh WM, Algra A, van Kooten F, et al. Magnesium sulfate in aneurysmal subarachnoid hemorrhage: A randomized controlled trial. *Stroke* 2005;36:1011–5.

15. Dorhout Mees SM, Algra A, Vandertop WP, et al. Magnesium for aneurysmal subarachnoid haemorrhage (MASH-2): A randomised placebo-controlled trial. *Lancet* 2012;380:44–9.

chapter nine

Magnesium deficiency in attention deficit hyperactivity disorder

Sanjay Singh, Mark Rabbat, Robert S. Dieter, Herbert Wilde, Alexandria N. Stockman, Elizabeth Rocha, Kiratipath Iamsakul, Raymond Dieter, Jasvinder Chawla, James Welsh, David Leehey, and Walter Jones

Contents

Causes and consequences of magnesium deficiency

Magnesium deficiency is rampant in the population for multiple reasons, among them:[1-21] *One*, decreased consumption of magnesium-rich foods such as green leafy vegetables grown in healthy mineral-rich soil that contains sufficient magnesium, zinc, iron, and other essential minerals typically depleted in over-farmed soil.[22-28] *Two*, overconsumption of *simple and easily digested complex carbohydrates* that deplete magnesium due to osmotic-diuretic effects. Even in healthy individuals *high glycemic load foods* can spike blood sugar sufficiently to cause acute diuresis and loss of magnesium,[14,29-31] but renal wasting of magnesium is particularly problematic in pre-diabetic and diabetic patients that have significant polyuria and polydipsia secondary to chronically elevated blood glucose levels.[4,5,7-10,14,16,20,30-38]

Three, vitamin D deficiency because vitamin D enhances magnesium absorption in the gut and 80% of the population in northern latitudes is vitamin D deficient.[14,29,39-51] *Four,* overconsumption of calcium in the modern diet, through supplementation and fortification, because calcium competes with magnesium for absorption in the gut.[49,52-56] In the ancient diet magnesium intake was significantly higher and calcium lower but trends have reversed; supplemental calcium is particularly problematic because it causes a sharp rise in blood calcium that augments its antagonism of magnesium.[19,44,49,52,53,55,57] *Five,* excess use of diuretics including alcohol, caffeine, and pharmaceuticals for hypertension because magnesium is one of the most water-soluble physiological electrolytes and rapidly depletes with diuresis.[17-19,58-64] Ironically, magnesium deficiency leads to increased vascular smooth muscle tone and pharmaceutical diuresis designed to lower blood pressure, through reductions in blood volume, contributes to hypertension through magnesium deficiency induced vasoconstriction.[35,61,65-74] *Six,* aerobic exercise and work in hot and humid environments deplete magnesium due to muscle activity and diaphoresis.[6,75-89] *Seven,* emotional, environmental, or physiological stress leads to sympathetic and adrenal activation and magnesium depletion that sensitizes the hypothalamic-pituitary-adrenal axis and increases sympathetic tone in a pathological positive feedback loop that further depletes magnesium (Table 9.1).[12,14,17,19,90-97]

Since magnesium is directly involved in all excitable cells, including smooth, cardiac, and skeletal muscle as well as neurons, is a co-factor in over 300 enzymes, and naturally antagonizes calcium, the physiological consequences of magnesium deficiency are ubiquitous and profound (Table 9.2).[5,6,12,14,17,19,20,35,49,57,60,68,73,92,98-100] Unfortunately, because magnesium deficiency develops insidiously the association between the multitude of magnesium deficiency symptoms with actual magnesium depletion are often missed.[6,14,17,19,33,99,101,102] To complicate matters, because *less than one percent* of body magnesium is in plasma and because plasma levels are tightly controlled by negative feedback loops and indirectly by endocrine mechanisms, including parathyroid hormone and calcitonin, clinical measurements of plasma magnesium can be misleading and mask magnesium deficiencies.[17,19,57,103-107] As plasma magnesium levels drop, magnesium *shifts from erythrocytes, soft tissue, and bone into the extracellular fluid* keeping plasma levels within a clinically "normal" range despite the fact that intracellular, tissue, and whole-body magnesium content may be substantially depleted.[6,14,104,107-110] Failure to recognize magnesium deficiency, because magnesium is not part of routine clinical blood work and because magnesium measurements can be misleading, may lead to treatment with multiple pharmaceuticals for each manifestation of the magnesium deficiency including arrhythmias, migraine, insomnia, or attention deficit hyperactivity disorder (ADHD).[98,99,111-116] Polypharmacia can lead to multiple drug-induced side effects but, most importantly, *pharmaceuticals only mask the underlying magnesium depletion* that can only be reversed

Table 9.1 Magnesium depleting and replenishing behaviors,
diets, and conditions[a]

Depleting diets and conditions	Replenishing diets and conditions
Excess Ethanol Consumption[b]	Green Leafy Vegetables Grown in Mineral-Rich Soil
Excess Aerobic Exercise[c]	Ocean Vegetables Rich in Minerals like Mg, I, & K
Activity in Hot & Humid Conditions, Diaphoresis	Consumption of Mineral Rich Nuts like Almonds
Acute Diuresis by High Glycemic Load Foods	Consumption of Well, Spring, or Hard Water
Chronic Diuresis of Prediabetes & Diabetes	Consumption of Vitamin D or Sun Exposure of Skin
Diuretics (Caffeine, Thiazides, Loop Diuretics)	Magnesium Supplementation
Calcium via Supplementation	Application of Topical Magnesium Oils & Creams
Certain Antibiotics: Amphotericin, Cyclosporine	Soaking in Epsom Salts or Certain Mineral Springs
Certain Oncotherapeutic Agents: Cisplatin	Stress Reduction Behaviors (Meditation, Massage)
Hyperthyroidism and Hyperparathyroidism	Renal Failure in Some Cases[e]
Sympathetic Overactivity	
Emotional or Physical Stress[d]	

[a] Incomplete List; For Reviews and Monographs See: Seelig,[14] Dean,[6] Torshin,[19] Vink,[102] Yardly,[17] Song,[17] Nishimuta,[161] Laires,[82] Altura,[99] Turner,[101] and Emoto[33]

[b] Threshold for how much alcohol is deleterious to magnesium levels depends on multiple variables including the subjects' liver health, height, weight, gender, and levels of alcohol dehydrogenase[58–60,161,224]

[c] Aerobic and strength training both deplete magnesium but exercise combined with profuse sweating deplete magnesium more rapidly; sweating alone depletes magnesium[18,75,80–84,86,87]

[d] Stress Includes: *Emotional*, such as fear, anger, sadness, or excitement; *Environmental*, like extreme heat, cold, restraint, imprisonment, loud sounds, or flashing lights; *Physical*, such as exercise, hunger, pain, injury, or illness; *Or, Physiological*, such as inflammatory or oxidative stress[12,14,19,90–97,256]

[e] Only contraindication for magnesium supplementation is renal failure due to inability of kidneys to clear magnesium; many with renal failure, though, are still magnesium deficient due to the use of diuretics, proton-pump inhibitors, and dialysis[2,3,48,153]

with dietary improvements, magnesium supplementation, and reduction of magnesium depleting behaviors such as excess exercise, excess alcohol and carbohydrate consumption, and excess stress.[5,79,17,19,32,33,38,59,60,75,81,82,84,87,89,111,117,118] Importantly and unlike with drugs, replenishing magnesium through diet and supplementation will not only resolve the primary condition for which the magnesium is being taken but also other conditions related to the

Table 9.2 Consequences of magnesium depletion[a]

Molecular and neuronal	Neurological and behavioral
Hypofunction of Na/K ATPase	ADD/ADHD
Increased NMDA Receptor Activation	Anxiety
Decreased Calcium Channel Inhibition	Irritability
Increased Intracellular Calcium	Inattention
Altered Potassium Channel Function	Migraine Headaches
Altered Neurotransmitter Release	Lower Threshold for Seizures
Increased Catecholamines	Compromised Memory
Increased Sympathetic Tone	Compromised Cognition
Reduced Parasympathetic Tone	Mania
Muscle Spasms and Muscle Cramps	Depression
Restless Leg Syndrome	Suicidal Ideation and Suicide

[a] Incomplete List; For Reviews and Monographs See: Seelig,[14] Dean,[6] Torshin,[19] Vink,[102] Song,[17] Nishimuta,[161] Laires,[82] Altura,[99] Turner,[101] and Emoto[33]

deficiency, many of which the patient and physician may be unaware are related to magnesium deficiency. For example, magnesium supplementation for premature ventricular contractions, an arrhythmia linked to magnesium deficiency, will also improve attention, reduce hyperactivity, improve sleep, and minimize migraines.[14,34,35,51,68,84,92,99,114,119–136]

Complications in magnesium research: Bioavailability and nutritional interactions

Much of the previous magnesium research is significantly compromised because the forms of magnesium used in these studies, mainly magnesium oxide or magnesium lactate, are *very poorly absorbed* compared to more bio-available forms or when magnesium is obtained from food; thus, *the presumed efficacy of magnesium based on these studies is a significant underestimate of the true efficacy of magnesium.*[127,129,130,135–147] Most studies that use magnesium oxide, or other poorly absorbed forms of magnesium, make no mention of the wide range of absorption characteristics of various magnesium formulations alluding to the lack of appreciation of this important variable.[127,129,130,135–138,140,141,145,146] Further, the poor absorption of magnesium oxide can lead to diarrhea and osmotic loss of magnesium and other electrolytes through the gut, a major concern in magnesium therapeutics that makes magnesium restoration with magnesium oxide impractical.[6,14,143,145,148–152] Consider the following: when supplementing with 400 mg of magnesium oxide only 240 mg of this is elemental magnesium and just 4%, or 10 mg, is absorbed while the rest serves to osmotically attract water into the gut, potentially leading to diarrhea and loss of magnesium and other electrolytes.[6,143,145–148,150,153] Importantly, studies of magnesium for ADHD rarely supplement with more than 400 mg of MgO to compensate for its poor absorption; yet, these studies draw conclusions about magnesium efficacy as if most of the magnesium in MgO is absorbed. In these studies, the bioavailability of the form of magnesium used is not discussed in light of the reported efficacy.[127,129,130,135,136,140,141,154–158] Second and third generation magnesium formulations that include chelates with various organic molecules, including glycine, lysine, malate, and citrate, have better absorption characteristics than MgO; however, in our decade-long experience with magnesium, bioavailability from these forms is not sufficient enough to adequately replenish magnesium in depleted individuals through oral supplementation alone.[137–139,142–147,150,151] The poor bioavailability of MgO may also explain why the efficacy of magnesium from *magnesium sulfate*, which is injected intravenously and bypasses the gut, is greater than with oral magnesium supplementation;[34,60,159,160] $MgSO_4$ must be injected intramuscularly or intravenously and is impractical for long-term daily supplementation.[160] Another important design flaw, with oral and particularly intravenous $MgSO_4$ studies, is that magnesium supplementation is only given for short durations. This is problematic because intracellular and tissue magnesium depletion and repletion have an unusually long time course, unlike any other electrolyte, except to a much lesser degree potassium, requiring months to years to fully restore.[6,14,15,17,19,148] This lag in repletion in soft tissue and bone contributes to underestimates of magnesium efficacy because with brief administration intracellular magnesium is only partially restored and recovery of function, therefore, is also partial.[6,14,15,19,106,148,149,161]

Many experts suggest the recommended dietary allowance for magnesium is too low for normal individuals but particularly low when factoring in age, as older individuals do not absorb magnesium as well, and considering other factors such as prediabetes, diabetes, exercise, and alcohol consumption, all of which significantly deplete magnesium.[5,9,14,16,32–35,38,59,62,84,162–165] To achieve symptomatic relief of magnesium deficiency symptoms, oral supplementation with magnesium oxide or most other magnesium formulations can be insufficient.[6,15,148,166–168] Fortunately, some newer magnesium supplements have much better bioavailability and include a well-absorbed form by Mega Foods (Manchester, New Hampshire; no financial disclosures), that has *an absorption and efficacy we estimate to be an order of magnitude greater* than other forms of magnesium including magnesium citrate. The enhanced absorption of the Mega Foods magnesium occurs, presumably, because it is extracted from plant sources and not synthesized or chelated to organic molecules like amino acids; even at relatively high doses, there are little or no laxative side effects, a primary concern in magnesium therapy. Carolyn Dean has developed a concentrated ionic solution of magnesium called ReMag™ that has a very good efficacy and little laxative side effects when consumed slowly.[148] Mechanisms of the differences in absorption properties of different forms of magnesium are unclear but an important area of magnesium research given the significant problems with magnesium absorption and bioavailability. Regardless of the form of magnesium used, topical application of magnesium is a good adjuvant to oral supplementation as the time frame to repletion of bodily stores is significantly faster than by oral supplementation alone.[15,166–168] Much of the previous research on magnesium has been conducted with low doses of poorly absorbed magnesium formulations without the addition of topical magnesium oils and lotions or greater amounts of magnesium to compensate for the poor absorption.[15,127,129,130,136,140,141,166–168] Despite these major flaws in previous magnesium research, overturning decades of published research, though flawed, can be a high-resistance path. Meanwhile, countless patients with undiagnosed magnesium deficiencies or those using poorly absorbed forms suffer from a *"magnesium deficiency syndrome"* that can include benign and lethal cardiac arrhythmias, recurrent migraines, insomnia, and inflammation in addition to inattention and hyperactivity.[6,7,14,17,19,32,33,35,61,95,99,102,106,114,128,148,169–173]

Apart from problems related to bioavailability of different magnesium formulations and the duration of administration, there are other reasons why the efficacy of magnesium supplementation in studies has been significantly underestimated. One important reason is that magnesium deficiencies rarely occur in isolation as they are usually a result of long-standing poor dietary habits and *magnesium deficiency is one variable in a larger equation of nutritional deficiencies that include other minerals, vitamins, and phytochemicals.*[40,41,46,49,51,127,133,135,141,174—177] Multiple lines of research suggest that subjects with ADHD are depleted not only of magnesium, but also zinc, iron, omega fatty acids, vitamin B6, and vitamin D.[40,41,46,47,49,51,127,133,135,141,174–176,178,179] These nutrients interact in synergistic ways; yet, most studies only test the efficacy of one nutrient in isolation. For example, studies of magnesium do not control for vitamin D levels even though vitamin D enhances absorption of magnesium in the gut and 80% of the population in northern latitudes is deficient.[44,46,47,49,51,178,179] Thus, studies in which magnesium is given in combination with 600–1000 IU of vitamin D should show greater efficacy than if magnesium were given alone. Ideally, the subject's entire diet should be improved with a focus on magnesium-rich terrestrial and ocean vegetables as well as other mineral rich foods including nuts and seeds; simultaneously, alcohol and starch consumption should be moderated. Although most appropriate for the subject and most effective in demonstrating the efficacy of nutritional therapy for multiple maladies, multiple variable-comprehensive nutritional change studies present their own set of challenges and the uncertainty of knowing what parts of the nutrient equation were responsible for the therapeutic efficacy is scientifically problematic. Further, it is impractical to blind subjects in comprehensive nutritional change studies. Clinical decisions, though, rely heavily on double-blinded, placebo-controlled studies as the "gold-standard" for altering evidence-based therapeutic algorithms and, thus, clinical decisions are inherently biased against comprehensive nutritional change studies where blinding the subject is impractical. The *one drug-one receptor paradigm* of typical pharmaceutical studies, however, is inappropriate for nutritional studies when one nutrient can potentially affect hundreds of different enzymes, channels, and genes and is itself affected by multiple other nutrients, phytochemicals, hormones, and physiological feedback loops.

Magnesium deficiency associated with attention deficit hyperactivity disorder

Studies that correlate magnesium levels with attention deficit disorder (ADD) and ADHD or use magnesium supplements to treat these disorders are *poorly done and have multiple research design flaws*, though there are notable exceptions.[127,129,130,135,136,140,141,155–158,174,180–182] Importantly, there are no large double-blind, placebo-controlled clinical trials that test well-absorbed forms of magnesium or large-scale studies that use micronutrient-dense vegetables and foods to treat ADD or ADHD. Evidence from such clinical trials is a prerequisite for evidence-based, nutritional approaches away from pharmaceuticals like methylphenidate (Ritalin) or dextroamphetamine (Adderall) that have significant cardiovascular and neural side effects including psychosis, mania, and tics in children.[112,113,115,116,183–192] Most existing studies of magnesium and ADHD suffer from small sample sizes and are often published in low-impact journals with less critical reviews.[127,129,130,135,136,140,141,155–158,174,180-182] Plasma magnesium measurements are used in most studies, which can be misleading, though a surprising number report magnesium levels in erythrocytes or hair, which are better indicators of total-body magnesium content than plasma (Table 9.3).[129,130,135,136,140,141,155–158,174,180–182] Invariably, the form of magnesium supplement used in these studies is one with poor bioavailability, usually magnesium oxide or magnesium lactate and, thus, only a small fraction of the ingested magnesium is absorbed.[127,129,130,135,136,140,155–158] Although some studies employ poly-nutrient therapy, adding vitamin B6, omega fatty acids, iron, or zinc to magnesium, none add vitamin D or measure vitamin D levels prior to magnesium supplementation.[127,129,130,155–158] Another problem with ADHD research, and magnesium and ADHD research in particular, is that treatment efficacy is often evaluated with *qualitative questionnaires* rather than *objective quantitative measures* like electroencephalograms   (EEG).[127,129,130,135,136,140,141,155–158,181,182,193–199]   Furthermore, symptoms of inattention and hyperactivity are associated with multiple heterogeneous causes including, in some, sensitivities to certain artificial

Table 9.3 Summary of studies on magnesium and ADD or ADHD

Age (years)	Sample size and controls (F/M)	Mg form and dose	Tissue measured	Primary findings
5–15	n = 249 (142/107)	---	Serum	Mg Low in 24/249; of these, 21/24 Had Inattention & "Neurotic Reactions"[182]
6–11	n = 51 n = 15	---	Plasma RBC[a]	Mg Low in Plasma & Erythrocytes of ADHD Subjects Compared to Controls[155]
18–24	n = 35 n = 112	---	Serum	Mg Higher in ADHD; OFA[b] Low in ADHD[174]
7.74 ± 1.48[c] 7.40 ± 1.35[c]	n = 20 (4/16) n = 20 (4/16)	---	Serum Hair	Mg, Zn, Cu Low in ADHD & Levels Correlate with Severity of ADHD Symptoms[141]
8.3 ± 1.8[c] 8.6 ± 3.1[c]	n = 58 n = 25	---	Serum	Mg, Zn, Fe Low in ADHD; Mg Similar in Inattention but Low in Hyperactive Subtype[181]
8.2 ± 0.60[c] 7.9 ± 0.87[c]	n = 9 (0/9) n = 11 (0/11)	---	Serum	Mg Similar to Controls but Higher During Stressful Venous Blood Collection[180]
6–12	n = 31 n = 20	Mg Lactate 96–144 mg/d	Plasma Eryth[a]	Mg Low in ADHD; Mg/Vit B6 (30 days) Increased Attention & Reduced Excitability & Anxiety[156-158]
0–15 "Mainly" 0–6	n = 52	Mg Lactate 6mg/kg/d	Serum Eryth[a]	Mg Low in 30/52 ADHD; Mg/Vit B6 (30–180 days) Decreased Excitability & Increased Attention[129]

(Continued)

Table 9.3 (Continued) Summary of studies on magnesium and ADD or ADHD

Age (years)	Sample size and controls (F/M)	Mg form and dose	Tissue measured	Primary findings
6.49[c] 4.37[c]	n = 40 (13/27) n = 36 (14/22)	Mg Lactate 6mg/kg/d	Serum Eryth[a]	Mg Low in ADHD; Mg/Vit B6 (60 or more days) Decreased Excitability & Increased Attention[130]
7–12	n = 50 n = 25	Mg[e] 200 mg/day	Serum, Hair Eryth[a]	Mg Low in ADHD & Mg (180 days) Reduces Excitability & Increases Attention[135,136]
7.74 ± 1.48[c] 7.40 ± 1.35[c]	n = 25 (5/20) n = 25 (6/19)	Mg[e] 200mg/d	Serum Hair	Mg Low in 18/25 ADHD Subjects; Mg (60 days) Decreased Excitability & Increased Attention[140]
5–12 8.6[d]	n = 810 (231/579)	Mg[e] 80mg/d	----	Mg, Zn, & OFA[b] (90 days) Decreased Excitability & Improved Attention[127]

[a] Erythrocytes or Red Blood Cells
[b] Omega Fatty Acids
[c] Mean ± Standard Deviation or Just Mean
[d] Median
[e] Magnesium Form Unspecified; Presumably Mg Oxide

food dyes and, in others, delays in development of the frontal lobes and reduced cortical thickness.[176,200–203] None of the magnesium and ADHD studies, though, exclude subjects with sensitivities to food dyes or measure frontal lobe cortical thickness prior to magnesium supplementation.[127,129,130,135,136,140,141,155–158,174,180–182] Inclusion of subjects with symptoms of inattention and hyperactivity *not primarily* due to magnesium and nutritional deficiencies will skew results suggesting magnesium is less efficacious than if exclusion criteria are more stringent.

In an early study, Nizankowska-Biaz et al. report significantly reduced levels of serum magnesium in 24 out of 249 children, aged 5 to 15, and that of those deficient in magnesium most had "neurotic reactions" and compromised attention (n = 21; Table 9.3).[182] Nogovitsina and Levitina find that hyperexcitable children, based on DSM-IV criteria (n = 51; aged 6 to 11) have reduced plasma and erythrocyte magnesium levels compared to controls (n = 15) and that supplementation with magnesium lactate and vitamin B6 restores plasma and erythrocyte magnesium, restores attention, reduces hyperexcitability, and improves EEG markers of ADHD.[155] The same authors later report that children given magnesium lactate and vitamin B6 (n = 31; aged 6 to 11) have decreased hyperexcitability, anxiety, and aggression and increased attention and erythrocyte magnesium levels.[156–158] Elbaz and colleagues report that Egyptian children diagnosed by DSM-IV criteria for ADHD (n = 20; aged 6 to 16) have levels of magnesium and zinc in hair that are significantly lower than in controls (n = 20) and levels correlate with severity of ADHD symptoms.[141] Mahmoud et al., in another study of Egyptian children, find that levels of magnesium in *serum* were lower in ADHD subjects diagnosed by DSM-IV criteria and Connor's Rating Scale (n = 58; aged 5 to 15) compared to age-matched controls (n = 25). Levels of magnesium in the inattentive subtype, though, do not differ significantly from levels in the hyperactive or combined subtypes of ADHD; zinc and ferritin levels were lower in all ADHD subtypes compared to controls.[181] Villagomez and Ramtekkar, in a review of magnesium and ADHD literature, conclude that magnesium, vitamin D, zinc, and iron levels are all low in ADHD subjects.[51] Surprisingly, Antalis et al. report that *serum magnesium levels are higher* in college-aged ADHD subjects (n = 35) than controls (n = 112); iron, zinc, and vitamin B6 are similar but omega-3 fatty acid levels are lower in ADHD subjects compared to controls.[174] Irmisch et al. find similar levels of magnesium in subjects with ADHD (n = 9) compared to controls (n = 11) when venous blood was collected under sedation, but higher in ADHD subjects when drawn under awake and more stressful conditions.[180] These unexpected results may be because plasma magnesium measurements are used in both studies and are poor indicators of true body-magnesium content. In the latter study, stress might lead to greater increases in plasma magnesium in some ADHD subjects with comorbid anxiety and increased response to stress.[90,94–96,204] Note also, the sample size in the Irmisch study is diminishingly small.[180] Interestingly, ADHD children have high resting heart rates and nighttime tachycardia[205] and hypomagnesemia is known to augment sympathetic activity to the heart and reduce vagal tone.[12,99,114,132,204–210] Thus, symptoms of inattention and hyperactivity and imbalances in autonomic control of the heart in ADHD subjects *may be manifestations of the same magnesium deficiency.* Although Adderall and Ritalin provide symptomatic relief of certain ADHD symptoms in some subjects by stimulating frontal lobe activity, they are amphetamines that increase catecholamine release and *augment sympathetic tone,* increase heart rate and blood pressure, and can induce psychosis, mania, and tics.[112,113,115,116,184–192] Magnesium should not only help resolve symptoms of ADHD, by mechanisms that are unclear, but magnesium will also *reduce* sympathetic tone, heart rate, and blood pressure.[20,35,65,68,74,92,99,114,127,129,130,135,136,140,141,156–158]

Magnesium supplementation for ADD and ADHD

Studies exist, in addition to those cited above, that use supplementation with magnesium for attention deficits and hyperactivity and further lend support to the magnesium and nutrition hypotheses of ADD and ADHD. Unfortunately, studies that supplement with magnesium to treat ADHD suffer from poor research design, small sample sizes, or use poorly absorbed forms of magnesium.[127,129,130,135,136,140,141,156–158] As with studies that correlate magnesium levels in plasma, erythrocytes, and hair, with ADHD, studies that use magnesium supplements for ADHD use outcome measures that are subjective and qualitative, which makes assessment of the efficacy of magnesium for ADHD more ambiguous.[127,129,130,135,136,140,141,156–158] In addition to standardized ADHD questionnaires, *objective quantitative measures like electroencephalographic changes in frontal lobe activity* should be included in the assessment of magnesium and nutritional therapy for attention deficits and hyperactivity.[193–199,211–216] Further, pilot studies and clinical trials of magnesium supplementation should exclude subjects who exercise excessively, drink alcohol in excess, or are pre-diabetic or diabetic because chronic loss of magnesium through muscle activity, diaphoresis, and diuresis, respectively, in these subjects will significantly attenuate the effects of oral magnesium supplementation and mask the true efficacy of magnesium.[5–10,14,17,19–21,29–33,35,38,59,60,62,75–78,80–85,87,217] Obviously, the most bioavailable form of magnesium should be given to subjects in future studies; however, there is no consensus in the magnesium research field which formulation is the most bioavailable as there are few systematic studies of magnesium bioavailability particularly of newer magnesium forms.[137–139,142–147,150,218] Much of the early magnesium research, in ADHD or otherwise, employed magnesium oxide or intravenous magnesium sulfate while newer studies use multiple different forms of magnesium with widely varying absorption characteristics. Variability in the forms used compromises comparisons across studies because the bioavailability of different forms can vary dramatically.[6,14,15,19,127,129,130,135,136,140,141,156–158] Plasma measurements of magnesium are misleading, but it is less certain what biospecimen is practical to biopsy and a good surrogate for whole-body magnesium content.[6,14,19,97,104–106,108,110,219] Particularly for clinical detection of occult *"magnesium deficiency syndrome"* in unsuspecting patients, it is imperative that these methods be standardized and made available ubiquitously in clinical environments.[97,104–106,108,110,219]

Starobrat-Hermelin and Kozielec gave children with ADHD (n = 50; aged 7 to 12) 200 mg of magnesium for 6 months and compared the effects to an age-matched control group (n = 25).[135,136] They measured magnesium levels in serum, red blood cells, and hair using atomic absorption spectroscopy and evaluated attention and hyperactivity using validated instruments including Conners Rating Scale for Parents and Teachers and the Wender-Utah Rating Scale.[135,136] After magnesium supplementation, *all measures of hyperactivity were significantly decreased, attention increased, and magnesium levels in hair concomitantly increased.*[135,136] Mousain-Bosc and colleagues report that erythrocyte magnesium is decreased in 30 out of 52 "hyperexcitable children," aged 15 and younger, and that 6 mg/kg/day magnesium lactate along with vitamin B6 restores erythrocyte magnesium in 4 to 24 weeks.[129] They also report that *symptoms of hyperexcitability, physical aggression, instability, inattention, and muscle spasms all decreased* when magnesium was given for 4 weeks or more using DSM-IV criteria for ADHD and Conners Rating Scale.[129] In a follow-up study, Mousain-Bosc et al. report that 6 mg/kg/day magnesium lactate with vitamin B6 given to children for 8 weeks or more (n = 40; aged 7 to 12) *reduced hyperactivity and increased attention*; erythrocyte magnesium levels increased significantly with supplementation.[130] Within 8 weeks of cessation of magnesium supplementation *hyperactivity and inattention symptoms reappeared.*[130] El Baza and colleagues found that ADHD subjects (n = 25; average age: 7.74 ± 1.48) given 200 mg/day magnesium showed significant decreases in hyperactivity and increases in attention compared to age-matched controls (n = 25; average age: 7.40 ± 1.35) using DSM-IV-R criteria for ADHD and Conners Rating Scale. Hair and serum magnesium levels increased with magnesium supplementation.[140] Huss and co-authors examined the behavior of children (n = 810; aged 5 to 12) after supplementation with magnesium (80 mg/day), omega fatty acids, and zinc, and found *improvements in attention and decreases in hyperactivity and impulsivity* after 12 weeks of therapy measured using standardized SNAP-IV evaluation scales.[127] Given the use of multiple supplements in some studies it is difficult to distinguish the effects of magnesium from that of zinc, omega fatty acids, vitamin B6, or iron; however, such poly-nutrient studies *in conjunction with exclusive mono-nutrient therapy studies* are essential to elucidate the role of magnesium and nutrition in ADHD.[127] Rucklidge et al. conclude that more research is needed before magnesium supplementation for ADHD can be recommended, though suggest evidence for the use of zinc in ADHD is more conclusive.[220] In another review, Hariri and Azadbakht state there is insufficient quality evidence to suggest use of magnesium, iron, or zinc in ADHD[175] whereas Sinn suggests that although omega-3 fatty acids for ADHD can be recommended, evidence for supplementation with magnesium is equivocal but likely due to poor bioavailability of forms used.[133]

Adult ADHD, prediabetes, and diabetes epidemic

ADHD has multiple variants but is commonly thought to be exclusive to children; adult ADD and ADHD, though, may be *among the most underdiagnosed psychiatric disorders* and concomitant with the prediabetes and diabetes epidemic may be present in unprecedented numbers.[221-223] Symptoms of adult ADD and ADHD can include "inattention, distractibility, restlessness, labile mood, quick temper, overactivity, disorganization, and impulsivity".[222-227] These symptoms are likely to be exacerbated after heavy aerobic exercise, significant stress, alcohol use, or after a high glycemic content meal particularly in prediabetics and diabetics.[4,5,7-10,18-21,32,33,35,38,58-60,62,64,75-77,81-85,87,88] In both adolescents and adults, ADHD is associated with obesity[35,221,228-231] that likely contributes to magnesium deficiency in at least two ways: *One,* overweight and obese individuals are less likely to have subsisted primarily on terrestrial and ocean vegetables rich in minerals and, thus, are likely to be magnesium deficient. *Two,* even modest amounts of visceral fat are associated with insulin resistance attenuating the insulin response to hyperglycemia.[5,7,8,20,32,33,232,233] As a consequence, in prediabetics and diabetics postprandial hyperglycemia after a carbohydrate-rich meal leads to increased renal plasma filtration and polyuria with, obligatory, osmotic wasting of magnesium and other minerals like potassium and zinc.[3,9,10,14,30,31,34,193,229] Prediabetics are often unaware of their condition and not clinically labeled as "prediabetics;" thus, they continue to consume high glycemic content foods that lead to hyperglycemia and an insulin surge resulting in mineral diuresis as well as inflammation.[6,14,17,19,102] If a diagnosis of adult ADD or ADHD is suspected, or other magnesium deficiency symptoms such as cardiac arrhythmias or migraines are present, then daily supplementation with a well-absorbed form of magnesium should help resolve these symptoms and, in the process, help confirm the magnesium deficiency as symptoms resolve.

Electroencephalographic markers
of ADD and ADHD

Electroencephalograms are useful non-invasive measures of brain electrical activity that correlate with changes in cortical activity and function. Based on the resolution of anatomical localization required, anywhere from less than 20 to more than 256 electrodes can be placed on the scalp in various configurations. Regardless of the spatial resolution achieved, EEG provides *very high temporal resolution of summed cortical synaptic potentials.*[234] Frequencies of cortical EEG activity can be subdivided into multiple bands that have *general* functional correlates: delta waves are less than 4 Hz and occur during deep sleep; theta waves are from 4 to 7 Hz and associated with drowsiness or reduced cortical activity; alpha waves occur during relaxed states and range from 8 to 13 Hz; beta waves are from 14 to 31 Hz and occur during alert and engaged states; gamma waves occur at frequencies beyond 31 Hz and are associated with interactions across different brain regions, though much about their origin remains mysterious.[194,234] ADHD subjects at all age groups have greater low-frequency theta activity and decreased beta in certain brain regions compared to controls; however, the extent of the reduced beta in ADHD subjects diminishes with age.[195,196] Based on these trends, Bresnahan et al. suggest that the differential changes in hyperactivity, which diminish with age, and impulsivity, which do not, that the decreased beta may be linked to hyperactivity and increased theta to impulsivity.[195] Bresnahan and Barry have also shown that adults with ADHD (n = 50) have elevated theta activity compared to controls (n = 50) and suggest that EEG is a *useful objective diagnostic tool for ADHD particularly in borderline subjects.*[196]

A review by Barry et al. of EEG in ADHD subjects also suggests that during resting conditions ADHD subjects have elevated relative theta power and reduced relative alpha and beta; further, ADHD subjects have increased theta/alpha and theta/beta *ratios compared to controls.*[194] These authors reinforce the fact that EEG is a useful diagnostic tool for ADHD and that despite the different ADHD subtypes certain EEG fingerprints persist across the entire spectrum of ADHD and through multiple developmental stages of ADHD.[194] Hobbs and colleagues found that ADHD subjects (n = 15) have greater absolute delta and theta and increased theta/beta ratios compared to controls (n = 15).[214] Bresnahan et al. report significant reductions in slow theta wave activity with dexamphetamine treatment in ADHD subjects (n = 50) to levels comparable to those of controls (n = 50).[211] Long-term use of stimulants, though, leads to deleterious cardiovascular consequences, including hypertension and tachycardia, and neural side effects including psychosis and mania in children;[112,113,115,183,185,188,191,192,235] treatment with more well-absorbed forms of magnesium should not only be effective for ADHD, as measured by psychometric and EEG markers, but magnesium actually offers cardiovascular benefits including reduced sympathetic and vascular tone and protection from benign and malignant arrhythmias.[12,61,68,99,114,173,204,209,236,237]

Resolution of ADHD symptoms with well-absorbed magnesium

Over the past decade, we have been treating college-aged and adult ADHD subjects, under our IRB approved protocol, with various forms of magnesium including magnesium oxide and magnesium citrate. Although our initial results with poorly absorbed forms of magnesium were positive, evaluated using DSM-V criteria for ADHD, Wender-Utah Scale, as well as EEG analysis of frontal lobe activity before and after magnesium supplementation, the results were less robust than anticipated based on existing literature. A breakthrough occurred when we started using a much better-absorbed form of magnesium from Mega Foods (400 mg/day; no financial disclosures) that led to consistent and unequivocal resolution of ADHD symptoms in each subject tested. As the study evolved through different stages, our exclusion criteria became more stringent with added exclusion of those self-reporting an alcohol history consistent with a DSM-V diagnosis of "alcohol use" or "alcohol abuse" disorder, those that exercise excessively, or those that are diabetic.[6,7,14,19,33,75–77,80–82,84,85,88,224] We find in college-aged students with pre-existing ADD or ADHD that a nutritional, alcohol, and exercise history is very telling whether they will respond to magnesium and nutritional therapy; in adults, whether they are *also pre-diabetic or diabetic foretells magnesium efficacy.*[5,35,58,59,62,75,80,81,84,96,110,117,238] It is unclear how much nutritional deficiencies versus delays in cortical development or sensitivities to food dyes and other unknown mechanisms contribute to the development of attention deficits and hyperactivity, though these causes likely overlap.[176,200,203,239–241] In our experience, every ADHD subject tested thus far has responded to magnesium therapy with improvements in attention and hyperactivity using either magnesium oxide or magnesium citrate (n = 15; aged 19 or more) and even more robustly with a well-absorbed form of magnesium from Mega Foods (n = 20; Manchester, NH). Electroencephalogram (EEG) analysis of subjects taking the Mega Foods magnesium (n = 10) reveals remarkable improvements in EEG markers of ADHD in these subjects *including reductions in frontal lobe theta activity*, indicating less frontal lobe hypofunction or *recovery of frontal lobe executive control*. Figures 9.1 and 9.2 show typical power spectra analysis of EEG recordings after supplementation with 400 mg of Mega Foods magnesium for 35 days in a 19-year-old male with significant ADHD symptoms prior to supplementation.[224,242] After magnesium supplementation, ADHD symptoms of inattention and hyperactivity *improved*

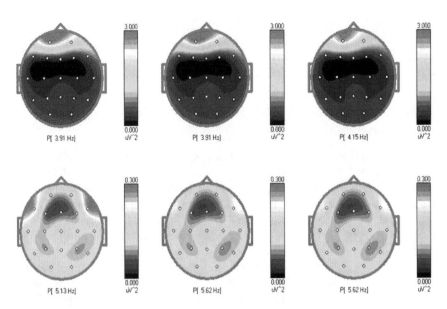

Figure 9.1 Power spectra analysis of electroencephalograms (EEG) of an ADHD subject before (top three panels) and after taking 400 mg/day of a well-absorbed form of magnesium from Mega Foods for 35 days (bottom three panels); this section of the recording occurred with the subject at rest and eyes closed. Significant reductions in frontal lobe theta (~4 to 8 Hz) occurred with magnesium supplementation represented by the decreased red in the frontal lobes after magnesium (bottom three panels). Note: the power scale for the lower panels is an order of magnitude smaller than for the upper panels reflecting dramatic reductions in theta activity. Concomitant with improvements in EEG markers of ADHD, the subjects ADHD symptoms including hyperactivity and inattention dramatically improved; academic and work performance also improved. One month after a "wash-out" period when magnesium supplementation was suspended symptoms of attention and hyperactivity returned. No other dietary or lifestyle changes were made during the study period.

dramatically along with improvements in EEG markers of ADHD. Self-reported social, academic, and employment performance also improved. After a washout period of one month, when magnesium supplementation was suspended, *symptoms of inattention and hyperactivity returned.*

For reasons that are unclear, there is an overlapping but dichotomous manifestation of ADHD and anxiety across genders with ADHD being more prevalent in boys and men and anxiety in girls and women, though significant numbers exist in each gender with comorbid anxiety and ADHD.[95,96,222,226,227,243–251] Recently, we have started treating subjects with anxiety disorder but without overt ADD or ADHD (n = 7; 300–400 mg/day) and the benefits from the Mega Foods magnesium have been

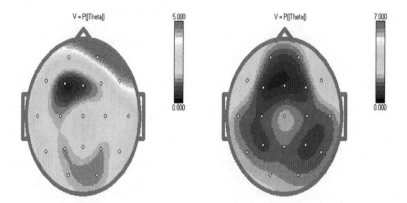

Figure 9.2 Power spectra analysis of EEG displaying summed average of full theta band activity (~4 to 8 Hz) for the same subject shown in Figure I before (left panel) and after (right panel) 400 mg of Mega Foods magnesium for 35 days. Dramatic reductions in theta activity occurred in the frontal lobes after magnesium supplementation represented by the reduced red in the frontal lobes after magnesium (right panel). Increased frontal lobe theta is a recognized EEG "fingerprint" in ADHD subjects and significant reduction after magnesium supplementation reflects return of frontal lobe-executive control over impulsivity and hyperactivity.[194–199,214,258]

remarkable in *substantially relieving their anxiety symptoms.* After a washout period of two weeks or more, with cessation of magnesium supplementation, *anxiety symptoms reappear.* Literature suggests there is a continuum of worsening symptoms that develop with increasing magnesium depletion where slight deficiencies lead to irritability, insomnia, and tachycardia, moderate deficiencies to anxiety, ADHD, and cardiac arrhythmias, and severe depletion contributes to mania, depression, and schizophrenia.[6,14,17,19,124,227,235,244,246,247,249,251–255] Some of the same research design flaws that exist in the magnesium and ADHD literature also exist in other areas of magnesium research including the use of poorly absorbed forms of magnesium and lack of large-scale clinical trials.[6,14,17,19,124,131,227,244,246,247,249,251–255] Although there is sufficient evidence based on the use of second and third generation magnesium formulations to warrant serious re-examination of the role of magnesium in ADD, ADHD, anxiety, sleep, and depression, overturning decades of research, though flawed, is a challenging prospect for modern magnesium researchers. Our findings, with much better-absorbed forms of magnesium than used in previous research, suggest that the efficacy of magnesium in ADD and ADHD has been grossly underestimated and suspect the same is true for the efficacy of magnesium for anxiety, sleep disorders, and depression.[95–97,121,122,124,149,248,256,257]

References

1. Al-Ghamdi SMG, Cameron EC, Sutton RAL. Magnesium deficiency: pathophysiologic and clinical overview. *Am. J. Kidney Dis.* 1994;24(5):737–752.
2. Alhosaini M, Walter JS, Singh S, Dieter RS, Hsieh A, Leehey DJ. Hypomagnesemia in hemodialysis patients: role of proton pump inhibitors. *Am. J. Nephrol.* 2014;39(3):204–209.
3. Alhosaini M, Leehey DJ. Magnesium and dialysis: the neglected cation. *Am. J. Kidney Dis.* 2015;66(3):523–531.
4. Blaszczyk U, Duda-Chodak A. Magnesium: its role in nutrition and carcinogenesis. *Rocz Panstw Zakl Hig.* 2013;64(3):165–171.
5. Chaudhary DP, Sharma R, Bansal DD. Implications of magnesium deficiency in type 2 diabetes: a review. *Biol. Trace Elem. Res.* 2010;134(2):119–129.
6. Dean C. *The Magnesium Miracle.* New York: Ballantine Books; 2007.
7. Guerrero-Romero F, Rodriguez-Moran M. Magnesium intake and the incidence of type 2 diabetes. In: Nishizawa Y, Morii H, Durlach J, eds. *New Perspectives in Magnesium Research.* London: Springer-Verlag; 2007:143–154.
8. Guerrero-Romero F, Bermudez-Pena C, Rodriguez-Moran M. Severe hypomagnesemia and low-grade inflammation in metabolic syndrome. *Magnes. Res.* 2011;24(2):45–53.
9. Hans CP, Sialy R, Bansal DD. Magnesium deficiency and diabetes mellitus. *Curr. Sci.* 2002;83(12):1456–1463.
10. Huerta MG, Roemmich JN, Kington ML, et al. Magnesium deficiency is associated with insulin resistance in obese children. *Diabetes Care.* 2005;28:1175–1181.
11. Nadler JL, Buchanan T, Natarajan R, Antonipillai I, Bergman R, Rude R. Magnesium deficiency produces insulin resistance and increased thromboxane synthesis. *Hypertension.* 1993;21:1024–1029.
12. Rayssiguier Y, Libako P, Nowacki W, Rock E. Magnesium deficiency and metabolic syndrome: stress and inflammation may reflect calcium activation. *Magnes. Res.* 2010;23(2):73–80.
13. Rude RK. Magnesium deficiency: a cause of heterogeneous disease in humans. *J. Bone Miner. Res.* 1998;13(4):749–758.
14. Seelig MS, Rosanoff A. *The Magnesium Factor.* New York: Avery; 2003.
15. Sircus M. *Transdermal Magnesium: A New Modality for the Maintenance of Health.* Bloomington, IN: iUniverse; 2011.
16. Sjogren A, Floren CH, Nilsson A. Magnesium deficiency in IDDM related to level of glycosylated hemoglobin. *Diabetes.* 1986;35:459–463.
17. Song Y. Magnesium intake, the metabolic syndrome, and chronic disease: a critical review of epidemiologic studies. In: Yardley AW, ed. *Dietary Magnesium: New Research.* New York: Nova Science Publishers; 2008:11–43.
18. Swales JD. Magnesium deficiency and diuretics. *BMJ.* 1982;285:1377–1378.
19. Torshin IY, Gromova OA. *Magnesium and Pyridoxine: Fundamental Studies and Clinical Practice.* New York: Nova Science Publishers; 2009.
20. Volpe SL. Magnesium in disease prevention and overall health. *Adv. Nutr.* 2013;4(3):378S–383S.
21. Volpe SL. Magnesium and the athlete. *Curr. Sports Med. Rep.* 2015;14(4):279–283.
22. Bennett WF. *Nutritional Deficiencies and Toxicities in Crop Plants.* Washington, DC: American Phythopathological Society Press; 1993.

23. Broadley MR, White PJ. Eats roots and leaves. Can edible horticultural crops address dietary calcium, magnesium and potassium deficiencies? *Proc. Nutr. Soc.* 2010;69(4):601–612.

24. Fan MS, Zhao FJ, Fairweather-Tait SJ, Poulton PR, Dunham SJ, McGrath SP. Evidence of decreasing mineral density in wheat grain over the last 160 years. *J. Trace Elem. Med. Biol.* 2008;22(4):315–324.

25. Graeft S, Steffens D, Schubert S. Use of reflectance measurements for the early detection of N, P, Mg and Fe deficiencies in *Zea mays L. J. Plant Nutr. Soil Sci.* 2001;164:445–450.

26. Guo W, Nazim H, Liang Z, Yang D. Magnesium deficiency in plants: an urgent problem. *Crop J.* 2016;4(2):83–91.

27. Hermans C, Verbruggen N. Enhancement of magnesium content in plants by exploiting ionomics and transcriptomics. In: Yardley AW, ed. *Dietary Magnesium: New Research.* New York: Nova Science Publishers; 2008:159–175.

28. Rosanoff A. Changing crop magnesium concentrations: impact on human health. *Plant Soil.* 2012;368 (1–2):139–153.

29. Gandhe MB, Jain K, Gandhe SM. Evaluation of 25(OH) vitamin D3 with reference to magnesium status and insulin resistance in T2DM. *J. Clin. Diagn. Res.* 2013;7(11):2438–2441.

30. Lopez-Alarcon M, Perichart-Perera O, Flores-Huerta S, et al. Excessive refined carbohydrates and scarce micronutrients intakes increase inflammatory mediators and insulin resistance in prepubertal and pubertal obese children independently of obesity. *Mediators Inflamm.* 2014;2014:849031.

31. Schwartz DL, Gilstad-Hayden K, Carroll-Scott A, et al. Energy drinks and youth self-reported hyperactivity/inattention symptoms. *Acad. Pediatr.* 2015;15(3):297–304.

32. Barbagallo M, Dominguez JL, Brucato V, et al. Magnesium metabolism in insulin resistance, metabolic syndrome, and type 2 diabetes mellitus. In: Nishizawa Y, Morii H, Durlach J, eds. *New Perspectives in Magnesium Research.* London: Springer-Verlag; 2007:213–223.

33. Emoto M, Nishizawa Y. Diabetes mellitus and magnesium. In: Nishizawa Y, Morii H, Durlach J, eds. *New Perspectives in Magnesium Research.* London: Springer-Verlag; 2007:197–212.

34. Geiger H, Wanner C. Magnesium in disease. *Clin. Kidney J.* 2012;5(Suppl 1):i25–i38.

35. Grober U, Schmidt J, Kisters K. Magnesium in prevention and therapy. *Nutrients.* 2015;7(9):8199–8226.

36. Mimouni F, Tsang RC, Hertzberg VS, Neumann V, Ellis K. Parathyroid hormone and calcitriol changes in normal and insulin-dependent diabetic pregnancies. *Obstet. Gynecol.* 1989;74(1):49–54.

37. Rotter I, Kosik-Bogacka D, Dolegowska B, Safranow K, Karakiewicz B, Laszczynska M. Relationship between serum magnesium concentration and metabolic and hormonal disorders in middle-aged and older men. *Magnes. Res.* 2015;28(3):99–107.

38. Sjogren A, Floren CH, Nilsson A. Magnesium, potassium and zinc deficiency in subjects with type II diabetes mellitus. *Acta. Med. Scand.* 1988;224:461–465.

39. Bener A, Ehlayel MS, Tulic MK, Hamid Q. Vitamin D deficiency as a strong predictor of asthma in children. *Int. Arch. Allergy Immunol.* 2012;157(2):168–175.

40. Bener A, Kamal M. Predict attention deficit hyperactivity disorder? Evidence-based medicine. *Glob. J. Health Sci.* 2014;6(2):47–57.

41. Bener A, Kamal M, Bener H, Bhugra D. Higher prevalence of iron deficiency as strong predictor of attention deficit hyperactivity disorder in children. *Ann. Med. Health Sci. Res.* 2014;4(Suppl 3):S291–297.
42. Farhanghi MA, Mahboob S, Ostadrahimi A. Obesity induced magnesium deficiency can be treated by vitamin D supplementation. *J. Pak. Med. Assoc.* 2009;59(4):258–261.
43. Goksugur SB, Tufan AE, Semiz M, et al. Vitamin D status in children with attention-deficit-hyperactivity disorder. *Pediatr. Int.* 2014;56(4):515–519.
44. Hardwick LL, Jones MR, Brautbar N, Lee DB. Magnesium absorption: mechanisms and the influence of vitamin D, calcium and phosphate. *J. Nutr.* 1991;121(1):13–23.
45. Hodgkinson A, Marshall DH, Nordin BE. Vitamin D and magnesium absorption in man. *Clin. Sci. (Lond).* 1979;57(1):121–123.
46. Kamal M, Bener A, Ehlayel MS. Is high prevalence of vitamin D deficiency a correlate for attention deficit hyperactivity disorder? *Atten. Defic. Hyperact. Disord.* 2014;6(2):73–78.
47. Krejs GJ, Nicar MJ, Zerwekh JE, Norman DA, Kane MG, Pak CY. Effect of 1,25-dihydroxyvitamin D3 on calcium and magnesium absorption in the healthy human jejunum and ileum. *Am. J. Med.* 1983;75(6):973–976.
48. Navarro JF, Mora-Fernandez C. Magnesium in chronic renal failure. In: Nishizawa Y, Morii H, Durlach J, eds. *New Perspectives in Magnesium Research*. London: Springer-Verlag; 2007:303–315.
49. Rosanoff A, Dai Q, Shapses SA. Essential nutrient interactions: does low or suboptimal magnesium status interact with vitamin D and/or calcium status? *Adv. Nutr.* 2016;7(1):25–43.
50. Schlingmann KP. Calcium-sensing receptor and magnesium. In: Nishizawa Y, Morii H, Durlach J, eds. *New Perspectives in Magnesium Research*. London: Springer-Verlag; 2007:272–285.
51. Villagomez A, Ramtekkar U. Iron, magnesium, vitamin D, and zinc deficiencies in children presenting with symptoms of attention-deficit/hyperactivity disorder. *Children (Basel).* 2014;1(3):261–279.
52. Behar J. Effect of calcium on magnesium absorption. *Am. J. Physiol.* 1975;229(6):1590–1595.
53. Care AD, Brown RC, Farrar AR, Pickard DW. Magnesium absorption from the digestive tract of sheep. *Q. J. Exp. Physiol.* 1984;69(3):577–587.
54. Hendrix ZJ, Alcock NW, Archibald RM. Competition between calcium, strontium, and magnesium for absorption in the isolated rat intestine. *Clin. Chem.* 1963;12:734–744.
55. Seelig MS. Increased need for magnesium with the use of combined oestrogen and calcium for osteoporosis treatment. *Magnes. Res.* 1990;3(3):197–215.
56. Watkins DW, Jahangeer S, Floor MK, Alabaster O. Magnesium and calcium absorption in Fischer-344 rats influenced by changes in dietary fibre (wheat bran), fat and calcium. *Magnes. Res.* 1992;5(1):15–21.
57. Hoorn EJ, Zietse R. Disorders of calcium and magnesium balance: a physiology-based approach. *Pediatr. Nephrol.* 2013;28(8):1195–1206.
58. Abbott L, Nadler J, Rude RK. Magnesium deficiency in alcoholism: possible contribution to osteoporosis and cardiovascular disease in alcoholics. *Alcohol Clin. Exp. Res.* 1994;18(5):1076–1082.
59. Flink EB. Magnesium deficiency in alcoholism. *Alcohol Clin. Exp. Res.* 1986;10(6):590–594.

60. Peake RW, Godber IM, Maguire D. The effect of magnesium administration on erythrocyte transketolase activity in alcoholic patients treated with thiamine. *Scott. Med. J.* 2013;58(3):139–142.
61. Seelig M. Cardiovascular consequences of magnesium deficiency and loss: pathogenesis, prevalence and manifestations--magnesium and chloride loss in refractory potassium repletion. *Am. J. Cardiol.* 1989;63(14):4G–21G.
62. Shane SR, Flink EB. Magnesium deficiency in alcohol addiction and withdrawal. *Magnes. Trace Elem.* 1991;10(2–4):263–268.
63. Sheehan JP, Seelig MS. Interactions of magnesium and potassium in the pathogenesis of cardiovascular disease. *Magnesium.* 1984;3(4–6):301–314.
64. Smets YF, Bokani N, de Meijer PH, Meinders AE. [Tetany due to excessive use of alcohol: a possible magnesium deficiency]. *Ned Tijdschr Geneeskd.* 2004;148(14):641–644.
65. Basrali F, Nasircilar Ulker S, Kocer G, et al. Effect of magnesium on vascular reactivity in NOS inhibition-induced hypertension. *Magnes. Res.* 2015;28(2):64–74.
66. Cengiz M, Ulker P, Uyuklu M, et al. Effect of magnesium supplementation on blood rheology in NOS inhibition-induced hypertension model. *Clin. Hemorheol. Microcirc.* 2016;63(1):57–67.
67. He L, Lang L, Li Y, Liu Q, Yao Y. Comparison of serum zinc, calcium, and magnesium concentrations in women with pregnancy-induced hypertension and healthy pregnant women: a meta-analysis. *Hypertens. Pregnancy.* 2016;35(2):202–209.
68. Houston M. The role of magnesium in hypertension and cardiovascular disease. *J. Clin. Hypertens. (Greenwich).* 2011;13(11):843–847.
69. Kh R, Khullar M, Kashyap M, Pandhi P, Uppal R. Effect of oral magnesium supplementation on blood pressure, platelet aggregation and calcium handling in deoxycorticosterone acetate induced hypertension in rats. *J. Hypertens.* 2000;18(7):919–926.
70. Kieboom BC, Stricker BH. Low serum magnesium is associated with hypertension. *J. Pediatr.* 2016;174:279–280.
71. Motoyama T, Sano H, Fukuzaki H. Oral magnesium supplementation in patients with essential hypertension. *Hypertension.* 1989;13(3):227–232.
72. Seelig CB. Magnesium deficiency in two hypertensive patient groups. *South. Med. J.* 1990;83(7):739–742.
73. Sontia B, Touyz RM. Role of magnesium in hypertension. *Arch. Biochem. Biophys.* 2007;458(1):33–39.
74. Sontia B, Touyz RM. Magnesium transport in hypertension. *Pathophysiology.* 2007;14(3–4):205–211.
75. Bohl CH, Volpe SL. Magnesium and exercise. *Crit. Rev. Food Sci. Nutr.* 2002;42(6):533–563.
76. Chen HY, Cheng FC, Pan HC, Hsu JC, Wang MF. Magnesium enhances exercise performance via increasing glucose availability in the blood, muscle, and brain during exercise. *PLoS One.* 2014;9(1):e85486.
77. Cordova A, Escanero JF, Gimenez M. Magnesium distribution in rats after maximal exercise in air and under hypoxic conditions. *Magnes. Res.* 1992;5(1):23–27.
78. Deuster PA, Dolev E, Kyle SB, Anderson RA, Schoomaker EB. Magnesium homeostasis during high-intensity anaerobic exercise in men. *J. Appl. Physiol. (1985).* 1987;62(2):545–550.

79. Golf SW, Happel O, Graef V, Seim KE. Plasma aldosterone, cortisol and electrolyte concentrations in physical exercise after magnesium supplementation. *J. Clin. Chem. Clin. Biochem.* 1984;22(11):717–721.

80. Konig D, Weinstock C, Keul J, Northoff H, Berg A. Zinc, iron, and magnesium status in athletes--influence on the regulation of exercise-induced stress and immune function. *Exerc. Immunol. Rev.* 1998;4:2–21.

81. Laires MJ, Monteiro C. Exercise, magnesium and immune function. *Magnes. Res.* 2008;21(2):92–96.

82. Laires MJ, Monteiro C. Exercise and magnesium. In: Nishizawa Y, Morii H, Durlach J, eds. *New Perspectives in Magnesium Research*. London: Springer-Verlag; 2007:173–185.

83. Lukaski HC, Nielsen FH. Dietary magnesium depletion affects metabolic responses during submaximal exercise in postmenopausal women. *J. Nutr.* 2002;132(5):930–935.

84. Nielsen FH, Lukaski HC. Update on the relationship between magnesium and exercise. *Magnes. Res.* 2006;19(3):180–189.

85. Soria M, Gonzalez-Haro C, Anson MA, Inigo C, Calvo ML, Escanero JF. Variations in serum magnesium and hormonal levels during incremental exercise. *Magnes. Res.* 2014;27(4):155–164.

86. Stark CM, Nylund CM, Gorman GH, Lechner BL. Primary renal magnesium wasting: an unusual clinical picture of exercise-induced symptoms. *Physiol. Rep.* 2016;4(8):e12773.

87. Terink R, Balvers MG, Hopman MT, Witkamp RF, Mensink M, Gunnewiek JM. Decrease in ionized and total magnesium blood concentrations in endurance athletes following an exercise bout restores within hours-potential consequences for monitoring and supplementation. *Int. J. Sport Nutr. Exerc. Metab.* 2016:1–22.

88. Tsiamis CB, Kakuris KK, Deogenov VA, Yerullis KB. Magnesium loss in magnesium deficient subjects with and without physical exercise during prolonged hypokinesia. *Clin. Invest. Med.* 2008;31(1):E16–23.

89. Veronese N, Berton L, Carraro S, et al. Effect of oral magnesium supplementation on physical performance in healthy elderly women involved in a weekly exercise program: a randomized controlled trial. *Am. J. Clin. Nutr.* 2014;100(3):974–981.

90. Allaert FA, Courau S, Forestier A. Effect of magnesium, probiotic, and vitamin food supplementation in healthy subjects with psychological stress and evaluation of a persistent effect after discontinuing intake. *Panminerva Med.* 2016;58(4):263–270.

91. Hans CP, Chaudhary DP, Bansal DD. Effect of magnesium supplementation on oxidative stress in alloxanic diabetic rats. *Magnes. Res.* 2003;16(1):13–19.

92. Johnson S. The multifaceted and widespread pathology of magnesium deficiency. *Med. Hypotheses.* 2001;56(2):163–170.

93. McCabe D, Colbeck M. The effectiveness of essential fatty acid, B vitamin, vitamin C, magnesium and zinc supplementation for managing stress in women: a systematic review protocol. *JBI Database System. Rev. Implement. Rep.* 2015;13(7):104–118.

94. Sartori SB, Whittle N, Hetzenauer A, Singewald N. Magnesium deficiency induces anxiety and HPA axis dysregulation: modulation by therapeutic drug treatment. *Neuropharmacology.* 2012;62(1):304–312.

95. Seelig MS. Consequences of magnesium deficiency on the enhancement of stress reactions; preventive and therapeutic implications (a review). *J. Am. Coll. Nutr.* 1994;13(5):429–446.
96. Serefko A, Szopa A, Poleszak E. Magnesium and depression. *Magnes. Res.* 2016;29(3):112–119.
97. Takase B, Akima T, Satomura K, et al. Effects of chronic sleep deprivation on autonomic activity by examining heart rate variability, plasma catecholamine, and intracellular magnesium levels. *Biomed. Pharmacother.* 2004;58(Suppl 1):S35–39.
98. Altura BM, Altura BT. Role of magnesium in patho-physiological processes and the clinical utility of magnesium ion selective electrodes. *Scand. J. Clin. Lab. Invest. Suppl.* 1996;224:211–234.
99. Altura BM, Altura BT. Magnesium: forgotten mineral in cardiovascular biology and atherogenesis. In: Nishizawa Y, Morii H, Durlach J, eds. *New Perspectives in Magnesium Research.* London: Springer-Verlag; 2007:239–260.
100. Seelig JM, Wei EP, Kontos HA, Choi SC, Becker DP. Effect of changes in magnesium ion concentration on cat cerebral arterioles. *Am. J. Physiol.* 1983;245(1):H22–26.
101. Turner JR, Vink R. Magnesium in the central nervous system. In: Nishizawa Y, Morii H, Durlach J, eds. *New Perspectives in Magnesium Research.* London: Springer-Verlag; 2007:338–355.
102. Vink R, Nechifor M, eds. *Magnesium in the Central Nervous System.* Adelaide, AU: University of Adelaide Press; 2011.
103. Dawson KG. Endocrine physiology of electrolyte metabolism. *Drugs.* 1984;28(Suppl 1):98–111.
104. Glasdam SM, Glasdam S, Peters GH. The importance of magnesium in the human body: a systematic literature review. *Adv. Clin. Chem.* 2016;73:169–193.
105. Mircetic RN, Dodig S, Raos M, Petres B, Cepelak I. Magnesium concentration in plasma, leukocytes and urine of children with intermittent asthma. *Clin.. Chim. Acta.* 2001;312(1–2):197–203.
106. Thomas J, Millot JM, Sebille S, et al. Free and total magnesium in lymphocytes of migraine patients – effect of magnesium-rich mineral water intake. *Clin. Chim. Acta.* 2000;295(1–2):63–75.
107. Waters RS, Fernholz K, Bryden NA, Anderson RA. Intravenous magnesium sulfate with and without EDTA as a magnesium load test-is magnesium deficiency widespread? *Biol. Trace Elem. Res.* 2008;124(3):243–250.
108. Arnaud MJ. Update on the assessment of magnesium status. *Br. J. Nutr.* 2008;99 (Suppl 3):S24–36.
109. Huijgen HJ, Soesan M, Sanders R, Mairuhu WM, Kesecioglu J, Sanders GT. Magnesium levels in critically ill patients. What should we measure? *Am. J. Clin. Pathol.* 2000;114(5):688–695.
110. Sanders GT, Huijgen HJ, Sanders R. Magnesium in disease: a review with special emphasis on the serum ionized magnesium. *Clin. Chem. Lab. Med.* 1999;37(11–12):1011–1033.
111. Dalsgaard S, Kvist AP, Leckman JF, Nielsen HS, Simonsen M. Cardiovascular safety of stimulants in children with attention-deficit/hyperactivity disorder: a nationwide prospective cohort study. *J. Child. Adolesc. Psychopharmacol.* 2014;24(6):302–310.

112. Hailpern SM, Egan BM, Lewis KD, et al. Blood pressure, heart rate, and CNS stimulant medication use in children with and without ADHD: analysis of NHANES data. *Front. Pediatr.* 2014;2:100.

113. Hammerness P, Wilens T, Mick E, et al. Cardiovascular effects of longer-term, high-dose OROS methylphenidate in adolescents with attention deficit hyperactivity disorder. *J. Pediatr.* 2009;155(1):84–89, 89.e1.

114. Hasebe N, Kikuchi K. Cardiovascular disease and magnesium. In: Nishizawa Y, Morii H, Durlach J, eds. *New Perspectives in Magnesium Research.* London: Springer-Verlag; 2007:227–238.

115. Samuels JA, Franco K, Wan F, Sorof JM. Effect of stimulants on 24-h ambulatory blood pressure in children with ADHD: a double-blind, randomized, cross-over trial. *Pediatr. Nephrol.* 2006;21(1):92–95.

116. Wilens TE, Hammerness PG, Biederman J, et al. Blood pressure changes associated with medication treatment of adults with attention-deficit/hyperactivity disorder. *J. Clin. Psychiatry.* 2005;66(2):253–259.

117. Durlach J, Collery P. Magnesium and potassium in diabetes and carbohydrate metabolism. Review of the present status and recent results. *Magnesium.* 1984;3(4–6):315–323.

118. Kisters K, Nguyen MQ, von Ehrlich B, Liebscher DH, Hausberg M. Low magnesium status and diabetes mellitus and hypertension. *Clin. Nephrol.* 2009;72(1):81–82.

119. Bianchi A, Salomone S, Caraci F, Pizza V, Bernardini R, D'Amato CC. Role of magnesium, coenzyme Q10, riboflavin, and vitamin B12 in migraine prophylaxis. *Vitam. Horm.* 2004;69:297–312.

120. Bobkowski W, Nowak A, Durlach J. The importance of magnesium status in the pathophysiology of mitral valve prolapse. *Magnes. Res.* 2005;18(1):35–52.

121. Chollet D, Franken P, Raffin Y, Malafosse A, Widmer J, Tafti M. Blood and brain magnesium in inbred mice and their correlation with sleep quality. *Am. J. Physiol. Regul. Integr. Comp. Physiol.* 2000;279(6):R2173–2178.

122. Chollet D, Franken P, Raffin Y, et al. Magnesium involvement in sleep: genetic and nutritional models. *Behav. Genet.* 2001;31(5):413–425.

123. Dhillon KS, Singh J, Lyall JS. A new horizon into the pathobiology, etiology and treatment of migraine. *Med. Hypotheses.* 2011;77(1):147–151.

124. Eby GA, Eby KL. Rapid recovery from major depression using magnesium treatment. *Med. Hypotheses.* 2006;67(2):362–370.

125. Gaul C, Diener HC, Danesch U, Migravent Study G. Improvement of migraine symptoms with a proprietary supplement containing riboflavin, magnesium and Q10: a randomized, placebo-controlled, double-blind, multicenter trial. *J. Headache. Pain.* 2015;16:516.

126. Hollifield JW. Potassium and magnesium abnormalities: diuretics and arrhythmias in hypertension. *Am. J. Med.* 1984;77(5A):28–32.

127. Huss M, Volp A, Stauss-Grabo M. Supplementation of polyunsaturated fatty acids, magnesium and zinc in children seeking medical advice for attention-deficit/hyperactivity problems - an observational cohort study. *Lipids Health Dis.* 2010;9:105.

128. Karamanli H, Kizilirmak D, Akgedik R, Bilgi M. Serum levels of magnesium and their relationship with CRP in patients with OSA. *Sleep and Breathing.* 2016; 21(2):549–556.

129. Mousain-Bosc M, Roche M, Rapin J, Bali JP. Magnesium VitB6 intake reduces central nervous system hyperexcitability in children. *J. Am. Coll. Nutr.* 2004;23(5):545S–548S.
130. Mousain-Bosc M, Roche M, Polge A, Pradal-Prat D, Rapin J, Bali JP. Improvement of neurobehavioral disorders in children supplemented with magnesium-vitamin B6. I. Attention deficit hyperactivity disorders. *Magnes. Res.* 2006;19(1):46–52.
131. Nielsen FH, Johnson LK, Zeng H. Magnesium supplementation improves indicators of low magnesium status and inflammatory stress in adults older than 51 years with poor quality sleep. *Magnes. Res.* 2010;23(4):158–168.
132. Omiya K, Akashi YJ, Yoneyama K, Osada N, Tanabe K, Miyake F. Heart-rate response to sympathetic nervous stimulation, exercise, and magnesium concentration in various sleep conditions. *Int. J. Sport Nutr. Exerc. Metab.* 2009;19(2):127–135.
133. Sinn N. Nutritional and dietary influences on attention deficit hyperactivity disorder. *Nutr. Rev.* 2008;66(10):558–568.
134. Somberg JC, Cao W, Cvetanovic I, Ranade VV, Molnar J. The effect of magnesium sulfate on action potential duration and cardiac arrhythmias. *Am. J. Ther.* 2005;12(3):218–222.
135. Starobrat-Hermelin B. [The effect of deficiency of selected bioelements on hyperactivity in children with certain specified mental disorders]. *Ann. Acad. Med. Stetin.* 1998;44:297–314.
136. Starobrat-Hermelin B, Kozielec T. The effects of magnesium physiological supplementation on hyperactivity in children with attention deficit hyperactivity disorder (ADHD). Positive response to magnesium oral loading test. *Magnes. Res.* 1997;10(2):149–156.
137. Coudray C, Rambeau M, Feillet-Coudray C, et al. Study of magnesium bioavailability from ten organic and inorganic Mg salts in Mg-depleted rats using a stable isotope approach. *Magnes. Res.* 2005;18(4):215–223.
138. Davenport GM, Boling JA, Gay N. Bioavailability of magnesium in beef cattle fed magnesium oxide or magnesium hydroxide. *J. Anim. Sci.* 1990;68(11):3765–3772.
139. Dolinska B, Ryszka F. Influence of salt form and concentration on the absorption of magnesium in rat small intestine. *Boll. Chim. Farm.* 2004;143(4):163–165.
140. El Baza F, AlShahawi HA, Zahra S, AbdelHakim RA. Magnesium supplementation in children with attention deficit hyperactivity disorder. *Egypt. J. Med. Hum. Genet.* 2016;17(1):63–70.
141. Elbaz F, Zahra S, Hanafy H. Magnesium, zinc and copper estimation in children with attention deficit hyperactivity disorder (ADHD). *Egypt. J. Med. Hum. Genet.* 2017;18(2):153–163.
142. Fine KD, Santa Ana CA, Porter JL, Fordtran JS. Intestinal absorption of magnesium from food and supplements. *J. Clin. Invest.* 1991;88(2):396–402.
143. Firoz M, Graber M. Bioavailability of US commercial magnesium preparations. *Magnes. Res.* 2001;14(4):257–262.
144. Hurley LA, Greene LW, Byers FM, Carstens GE. Site and extent of apparent magnesium absorption by lambs fed different sources of magnesium. *J. Anim. Sci.* 1990;68(8):2181–2187.
145. Lindberg JS, Zobitz MM, Poindexter JR, Pak CY. Magnesium bioavailability from magnesium citrate and magnesium oxide. *J. Am. Coll. Nutr.* 1990;9(1):48–55.

146. Schuette SA, Lashner BA, Janghorbani M. Bioavailability of magnesium diglycinate vs magnesium oxide in patients with ileal resection. *JPEN J. Parenter. Enteral. Nutr.* 1994;18(5):430–435.

147. Walker AF, Marakis G, Christie S, Byng M. Mg citrate found more bioavailable than other Mg preparations in a randomised, double-blind study. *Magnes. Res.* 2003;16(3):183–191.

148. Dean C. *Invisible Minerals: The Pico-Ionic Magnesium Solution.* Kindle: Amazon Digital Services; 2013.

149. De Souza MC, Walker AF, Robinson PA, Bolland K. A synergistic effect of a daily supplement for 1 month of 200 mg magnesium plus 50 mg vitamin B6 for the relief of anxiety-related premenstrual symptoms: a randomized, double-blind, crossover study. *J. Women's Health Gend. Based Med.* 2000;9(2):131–139.

150. Siener R, Jahnen A, Hesse A. Bioavailability of magnesium from different pharmaceutical formulations. *Urol. Res.* 2011;39(2):123–127.

151. Spasov AA, Petrov VI, Iezhitsa IN, Kravchenko MS, Kharitonova MV, Ozerov AA. [Comparative study of magnesium salts bioavailability in rats fed a magnesium-deficient diet]. *Vestn Ross Akad Med Nauk.* 2010(2):29–37.

152. Yoshimura Y, Fujisaki K, Yamamoto T, Shinohara Y. Pharmacokinetic studies of orally administered magnesium oxide in rats. *Yakugaku Zasshi.* 2017;137(5):581–587.

153. Durlach J, Durlach V, Bac P, Bara M, Guiet-Bara A. Magnesium and therapeutics. *Magnes. Res.* 1994;7(3–4):313–328.

154. Maor NR, Alperin M, Shturman E, et al. Effect of magnesium oxide supplementation on nocturnal leg cramps: a randomized clinical trial. *JAMA Intern. Med.* 2017;177(5):617–623.

155. Nogovitsina OR, Levitina EV. [Diagnostic value of examination of the magnesium homeostasis in children with attention deficit syndrome with hyperactivity]. *Klin Lab Diagn.* 2005(5):17–19.

156. Nogovitsina OR, Levitina EV. [Effect of MAGNE-B6 on the clinical and biochemical manifestations of the syndrome of attention deficit and hyperactivity in children]. *Eksp Klin Farmakol.* 2006;69(1):74–77.

157. Nogovitsina OR, Levitina EV. [Neurological aspect of clinical symptoms, pathophysiology and correction in attention deficit hyperactivity disorder]. *Zh Nevrol Psikhiatr Im S S Korsakova.* 2006;106(2):17–20.

158. Nogovitsina OR, Levitina EV. Neurological aspects of the clinical features, pathophysiology, and corrections of impairments in attention deficit hyperactivity disorder. *Neurosci. Behav. Physiol.* 2007;37(3):199–202.

159. Reed BN, Zhang S, Marron JS, Montague D. Comparison of intravenous and oral magnesium replacement in hospitalized patients with cardiovascular disease. *Am. J. Health. Syst. Pharm.* 2012;69(14):1212–1217.

160. Saha PK, Kaur J, Goel P, Kataria S, Tandon R, Saha L. Safety and efficacy of low dose intramuscular magnesium sulphate (MgSO4) compared to intravenous regimen for treatment of eclampsia. *J. Obstet. Gynaecol. Res.* 2017;43(10):1543–1549.

161. Nishimuta M, Kodama N, Morikuni E, et al. Magnesium requirements and affecting factors. In: Nishizawa Y, Morii H, Durlach J, eds. *New Perspectives in Magnesium Research.* London: Springer-Verlag; 2007:94–102.

162. Bergman C, Gray-Scott D, Chen JJ, Meacham S. What is next for the Dietary Reference Intakes for bone metabolism related nutrients beyond calcium: phosphorus, magnesium, vitamin D, and fluoride? *Crit. Rev. Food Sci. Nutr.* 2009;49(2):136–144.

163. Durlach J. Recommended dietary amounts of magnesium: Mg RDA. *Magnes. Res.* 1989;2(3):195–203.

164. Ouchi Y, Orimo H. [Calcium and magnesium metabolism in the aged]. *Nihon Ronen Igakkai Zasshi.* 1989;26(3):216–222.

165. Vaquero MP. Magnesium and trace elements in the elderly: intake, status and recommendations. *J. Nutr. Health Aging.* 2002;6(2):147–153.

166. Chandrasekaran NC, Sanchez WY, Mohammed YH, Grice JE, Roberts MS, Barnard RT. Permeation of topically applied Magnesium ions through human skin is facilitated by hair follicles. *Magnes. Res.* 2016;29(2):35–42.

167. Engen DJ, McAllister SJ, Whipple MO, et al. Effects of transdermal magnesium chloride on quality of life for patients with fibromyalgia: a feasibility study. *J. Integr. Med.* 2015;13(5):306–313.

168. Kass L, Rosanoff A, Tanner A, Sullivan K, McAuley W, Plesset M. Effect of transdermal magnesium cream on serum and urinary magnesium levels in humans: a pilot study. *PLoS One.* 2017;12(4):e0174817.

169. Martin BR, Seaman DR. Dietary and lifestyle changes in the treatment of a 23-year-old female patient with migraine. *J. Chiropr. Med.* 2015;14(3):205–211.

170. Mauskop A, Altura BT, Cracco RQ, Altura BM. Deficiency in serum ionized magnesium but not total magnesium in patients with migraines. Possible role of ICa2+/IMg2+ ratio. *Headache.* 1993;33:135–138.

171. Merison K, Jacobs H. Diagnosis and treatment of childhood migraine. *Curr. Treat. Options Neurol.* 2016;18(11):48.

172. Ondo WG. Restless legs syndrome. *Neurol. Clin.* 2009;27(3):779–799, vii.

173. Seelig MS. Interrelationship of magnesium and congestive heart failure. *Wien Med Wochenschr.* 2000;150(15–16):335–341.

174. Antalis CJ, Stevens LJ, Campbell M, Pazdro R, Ericson K, Burgess JR. Omega-3 fatty acid status in attention-deficit/hyperactivity disorder. *Prostaglandins Leukot Essent Fatty Acids.* 2006;75(4–5):299–308.

175. Hariri M, Azadbakht L. Magnesium, iron, and zinc supplementation for the treatment of attention deficit hyperactivity disorder: a systematic review on the recent literature. *Int. J. Prev. Med.* 2015;6:83.

176. Konikowska K, Regulska-Ilow B, Rozanska D. The influence of components of diet on the symptoms of ADHD in children. *Rocz Panstw Zakl Hig.* 2012;63(2):127–134.

177. Chawla J, Kvarnberg D. Hydrosoluble vitamins. *Handb. Clin. Neurol.* 2014;120:891–914.

178. Deng X, Song Y, Manson JE, et al. Magnesium, vitamin D status and mortality: results from US National Health and Nutrition Examination Survey (NHANES) 2001 to 2006 and NHANES III. *BMC Med.* 2013;11:187.

179. Pointillart A, Denis I, Colin C. Effects of dietary vitamin D on magnesium absorption and bone mineral contents in pigs on normal magnesium intakes. *Magnes. Res.* 1995;8(1):19–26.

180. Irmisch G, Thome J, Reis O, Hassler F, Weirich S. Modified magnesium and lipoproteins in children with attention deficit hyperactivity disorder (ADHD). *World J. Biol. Psychiatry.* 2011;12(Suppl 1):63–65.

181. Mahmoud MM, El-Mazary AA, Maher RM, Saber MM. Zinc, ferritin, magnesium and copper in a group of Egyptian children with attention deficit hyperactivity disorder. *Ital. J. Pediatr.* 2011;37:60.

182. Nizankowska-Blaz T, Korczowski R, Zys K, Rybak A. [Level of magnesium in blood serum in children from the province of Rzesz'ow]. *Wiad Lek.* 1993;46(3–4):120–122.

183. Belanger SA, Warren AE, Hamilton RM, et al. Cardiac risk assessment before the use of stimulant medications in children and youth. *Paediatr. Child Health.* 2009;14(9):579–592.

184. Buchhorn R, Christian W. Ventricular arrhythmias in children with attention deficit disorder--a symptom of autonomic imbalance? *Cardiol. Young.* 2014;24(1):120–125.

185. Cherland E, Fitzpatrick R. Psychotic side effects of psychostimulants: a 5-year review. *Can. J. Psychiatry.* 1999;44:811–813.

186. Findling RL, Dogin JW. Psychopharmacology of ADHD: children and adolescents. *J. Clin. Psychiatry.* 1998;59 (Suppl 7):42–49.

187. Kosse RC, Bouvy ML, Philbert D, de Vries TW, Koster ES. Attention-deficit/hyperactivity disorder medication use in adolescents: the patient's perspective. *J. Adolesc. Health.* 2017;61(5):619–625.

188. Lakhan SE, Kirchgessner A. Prescription stimulants in individuals with and without attention deficit hyperactivity disorder: misuse, cognitive impact, and adverse effects. *Brain Behav.* 2012;2(5):661–677.

189. Matsudaira T. Attention deficit disorders--drugs or nutrition? *Nutr. Health.* 2007;19(1–2):57–60.

190. Monastra VJ, Monastra DM, George S. The effects of stimulant therapy, EEG biofeedback, and parenting style on the primary symptoms of attention-deficit/hyperactivity disorder. *Appl. Psychophysiol. Biofeedback.* 2002;27(4):231–249.

191. Ross RG. Psychotic and manic-like symptoms during stimulant treatment of attention deficit hyperactivity disorder. *Am. J. Psychiatry.* 2006;163(7):1149–1152.

192. Varley CK, Vincent J, Varley P, Calderon R. Emergence of tics in children with attention deficit hyperactivity disorder treated with stimulant medications. *Compr. Psychiatry.* 2001;42(3):228–233.

193. Alba G, Pereda E, Manas S, Mendez LD, Gonzalez A, Gonzalez JJ. Electroencephalography signatures of attention-deficit/hyperactivity disorder: clinical utility. *Neuropsychiatr. Dis. Treat.* 2015;11:2755–2769.

194. Barry RJ, Clarke AR, Johnstone SJ. A review of electrophysiology in attention-deficit/hyperactivity disorder: I. Qualitative and quantitative electroencephalography. *Clin. Neurophysiol.* 2003;114(2):171–183.

195. Bresnahan SM, Anderson JW, Barry RJ. Age-related changes in quantitative EEG in attention-deficit/hyperactivity disorder. *Biol Psychiatry.* 1999;46(12):1690–1697.

196. Bresnahan SM, Barry RJ. Specificity of quantitative EEG analysis in adults with attention deficit hyperactivity disorder. *Psychiatry. Res.* 2002;112(2):133–144.

197. Kamida A, Shimabayashi K, Oguri M, et al. EEG power spectrum analysis in children with ADHD. *Yonago Acta Medica.* 2016;59:169–173.

198. Markovska-Simoska S, Pop-Jordanova N. Quantitative EEG in children and adults with attention deficit hyperactivity disorder: comparison of absolute and relative power spectra and theta/beta ratio. *Clin. EEG Neurosci.* 2017;48(1):20–32.
199. Swatzyna RJ, Tarnow JD, Roark A, Mardick J. The utility of EEG in attention deficit hyperactivity disorder: a replication study. *Clin. EEG Neurosci.* 2017;48(4):243–245.
200. Arnold LE, Lofthouse N, Hurt E. Artificial food colors and attention-deficit/hyperactivity symptoms: conclusions to dye for. *Neurotherapeutics.* 2012;9(3):599–609.
201. Hesslinger B, Tebartz van Elst L, Thiel T, Haegele K, Hennig J, Ebert D. Frontoorbital volume reductions in adult patients with attention deficit hyperactivity disorder. *Neurosci. Lett.* 2002;328(3):319–321.
202. Millichap JG, Yee MM. The diet factor in attention-deficit/hyperactivity disorder. *Pediatrics.* 2012;129(2):330–337.
203. Mostofsky SH, Cooper KL, Kates WR, Denckla MB, Kaufmann WE. Smaller prefrontal and premotor volumes in boys with attention-deficit/hyperactivity disorder. *Biol. Psychiatry.* 2002;52(8):785–794.
204. Wienecke E, Nolden C. [Long-term HRV analysis shows stress reduction by magnesium intake]. *MMW Fortschr. Med.* 2016;158(Suppl 6):12–16.
205. Imeraj L, Antrop I, Roeyers H, Deschepper E, Bal S, Deboutte D. Diurnal variations in arousal: a naturalistic heart rate study in children with ADHD. *Eur. Child Adolesc. Psychiatry.* 2011;20(8):381–392.
206. Beauchaine TP, Gatzke-Kopp L, Neuhaus E, Chipman J, Reid MJ, Webster-Stratton C. Sympathetic- and parasympathetic-linked cardiac function and prediction of externalizing behavior, emotion regulation, and prosocial behavior among preschoolers treated for ADHD. *J. Consult. Clin. Psychol.* 2013;81(3):481–493.
207. Das UN. Nutritional factors in the pathobiology of human essential hypertension. *Nutrition.* 2001;17(4):337–346.
208. Musser ED, Backs RW, Schmitt CF, Ablow JC, Measelle JR, Nigg JT. Emotion regulation via the autonomic nervous system in children with attention-deficit/hyperactivity disorder (ADHD). *J. Abnorm. Child Psychol.* 2011;39(6):841–852.
209. Peeters E, Neyt A, Beckers F, De Smet S, Aubert AE, Geers R. Influence of supplemental magnesium, tryptophan, vitamin C, and vitamin E on stress responses of pigs to vibration. *J. Anim. Sci.* 2005;83(7):1568–1580.
210. Singh RB, Pella D, Neki NS, et al. Mechanisms of acute myocardial infarction study (MAMIS). *Biomed. Pharmacother.* 2004;58(Suppl 1):S111–115.
211. Bresnahan SM, Barry RJ, Clarke AR, Johnstone SJ. Quantitative EEG analysis in dexamphetamine-responsive adults with attention-deficit/hyperactivity disorder. *Psychiatry. Res.* 2006;141(2):151–159.
212. Clarke AR, Barry RJ, Baker IE, McCarthy R, Selikowitz M. An investigation of stimulant effects on the EEG of children with attention-deficit/hyperactivity disorder. *Clin. EEG Neurosci.* 2017;48(4):235–242.
213. Hasler R, Perroud N, Meziane HB, et al. Attention-related EEG markers in adult ADHD. *Neuropsychologia.* 2016;87:120–133.
214. Hobbs MJ, Clarke AR, Barry RJ, McCarthy R, Selikowitz M. EEG abnormalities in adolescent males with AD/HD. *Clin. Neurophysiol.* 2007;118(2):363–371.

215. Rodriguez C, Gonzalez-Castro P, Cueli M, Areces D, Gonzalez-Pienda JA. Attention deficit/hyperactivity disorder (ADHD) diagnosis: an activation-executive model. *Front. Psychol.* 2016;7:1406.

216. Woltering S, Jung J, Liu Z, Tannock R. Resting state EEG oscillatory power differences in ADHD college students and their peers. *Behav. Brain. Funct.* 2012;8:60.

217. Lukaski HC. Vitamin and mineral status: effects on physical performance. *Nutrition.* 2004;20(7–8):632–644.

218. Bertinato J, Plouffe LJ, Lavergne C, Ly C. Bioavailability of magnesium from inorganic and organic compounds is similar in rats fed a high phytic acid diet. *Magnes. Res.* 2014;27(4):175–185.

219. Rude RK, Kirchen ME, Gruber HE, Meyer MH, Luck JS, Crawford DL. Magnesium deficiency-induced osteoporosis in the rat: uncoupling of bone formation and bone resorption. *Magnes. Res.* 1999;12(4):257–267.

220. Rucklidge JJ, Johnstone J, Kaplan BJ. Nutrient supplementation approaches in the treatment of ADHD. *Expert. Rev. Neurother.* 2009;9(4):461–476.

221. Chen HJ, Lee YJ, Yeh GC, Lin HC. Association of attention-deficit/hyperactivity disorder with diabetes: a population-based study. *Pediatr. Res.* 2013;73(4 Pt. 1):492–496.

222. Faraone SV, Biederman J, Spencer T, et al. Attention-deficit/hyperactivity disorder in adults: an overview. *Biol. Psychiatry.* 2000;48(1):9–20.

223. Wender PH. Attention-deficit hyperactivity disorder in adults. *Psychiatr. Clin. North. Am.* 1998;21(4):761–774, v.

224. American Psychiatric Association. *Diagnostic and Statistical Manual of Mental Disorders, DSM-5.* 5th ed. Washington, DC: American Psychiatric Association; 2013.

225. Chandler ML. Psychotherapy for adult attention deficit/hyperactivity disorder: a comparison with cognitive behaviour therapy. *J. Psychiatr. Ment. Health Nurs.* 2013;20(9):814–820.

226. Noren Selinus E, Molero Y, Lichtenstein P, et al. Subthreshold and threshold attention deficit hyperactivity disorder symptoms in childhood: psychosocial outcomes in adolescence in boys and girls. *Acta. Psychiatr. Scand.* 2016;134(6):533–545.

227. Xia W, Shen L, Zhang J. Comorbid anxiety and depression in school-aged children with attention deficit hyperactivity disorder (ADHD) and selfreported symptoms of ADHD, anxiety, and depression among parents of school-aged children with and without ADHD. *Shanghai Arch. Psychiatry.* 2015;27(6):356–367.

228. Fuemmeler BF, Ostbye T, Yang C, McClernon FJ, Kollins SH. Association between attention-deficit/hyperactivity disorder symptoms and obesity and hypertension in early adulthood: a population-based study. *Int. J. Obes. (Lond).* 2011;35(6):852–862.

229. Johnson RJ, Gold MS, Johnson DR, et al. Attention-deficit/hyperactivity disorder: is it time to reappraise the role of sugar consumption? *Postgrad. Med.* 2011;123(5):39–49.

230. Kountouris D, Bougioukou A, Koutsobelis K, Karachristou K. CBP023 Is there a correlation between attention deficit/hyperactivity disorder (ADHD) and obesity in children? *Eur. J. Paediatr. Neurol.* 2007;11:92.

231. Pagoto SL, Curtin C, Lemon SC, et al. Association between adult attention deficit/hyperactivity disorder and obesity in the US population. *Obesity (Silver Spring).* 2009;17(3):539–544.

232. Laires MJ, Moreira H, Monteiro CP, et al. Magnesium, insulin resistance and body composition in healthy postmenopausal women. *J. Am. Coll. Nutr.* 2004;23(5):510S–513S.

233. Zhang M, Hu T, Zhang S, Zhou L. Associations of different adipose tissue depots with insulin resistance: a systematic review and meta-analysis of observational studies. *Sci. Rep.* 2015;5:18495.

234. Fisch B. *Fisch and Spehlmann's EEG Primer: Basic Principles of Digital and Analog EEG.* 3rd ed. San Diego, CA: Elsevier Health Sciences; 2000.

235. Barbosa FJ, Hesse B, de Almeida RB, Baretta IP, Boerngen-Lacerda R, Andreatini R. Magnesium sulfate and sodium valproate block methylphenidate-induced hyperlocomotion, an animal model of mania. *Pharmacol. Rep.* 2011;63(1):64–70.

236. Rosanoff A. The high heart health value of drinking-water magnesium. *Med. Hypotheses.* 2013;81(6):1063–1065.

237. Spasov AA, Iezhitsa IN, Kharitonova MV, Gurova NA. Arrhythmogenic threshold of the myocardium under conditions of magnesium deficiency. *Bull. Exp. Biol. Med.* 2008;146(1):63–65.

238. Kaur B, Henry J. Micronutrient status in type 2 diabetes: a review. *Adv. Food. Nutr. Res.* 2014;71:55–100.

239. Seidman LJ, Valera EM, Makris N. Structural brain imaging of attention-deficit/hyperactivity disorder. *Biol. Psychiatry.* 2005;57(11):1263–1272.

240. Shaw P, Gornick M, Lerch J, et al. Polymorphisms of the dopamine D4 receptor, clinical outcome, and cortical structure in attention-deficit/hyperactivity disorder. *Arch. Gen. Psychiatry.* 2007;64(8):921–931.

241. Shaw P, Eckstrand K, Sharp W, et al. Attention-deficit/hyperactivity disorder is characterized by a delay in cortical maturation. *Proc. Natl. Acad. Sci. U.S.A.* 2007;104(49):19649–19654.

242. Ward MF, Wender PH, Reimherr FW. The Wender Utah Rating Scale: an aid in the retrospective diagnosis of childhood attention deficit hyperactivity disorder. *Am. J Psychiatry.* 1993;150(6):885–890.

243. Bron TI, Bijlenga D, Verduijn J, Penninx BW, Beekman AT, Kooij JJ. Prevalence of ADHD symptoms across clinical stages of major depressive disorder. *J. Affect. Disord.* 2016;197:29–35.

244. Ghanizadeh A. Predictors of different types of developmental coordination problems in ADHD: the effect of age, gender, ADHD symptom severity and comorbidities. *Neuropediatrics.* 2010;41(4):176–181.

245. Jarrett MA, Ollendick TH. A conceptual review of the comorbidity of attention-deficit/hyperactivity disorder and anxiety: implications for future research and practice. *Clin. Psychol. Rev.* 2008;28(7):1266–1280.

246. Kessler RC, Adler LA, Barkley R, et al. Patterns and predictors of attention-deficit/hyperactivity disorder persistence into adulthood: results from the national comorbidity survey replication. *Biol. Psychiatry.* 2005;57(11):1442–1451.

247. Mick E, Spencer T, Wozniak J, Biederman J. Heterogeneity of irritability in attention-deficit/hyperactivity disorder subjects with and without mood disorders. *Biol. Psychiatry.* 2005;58(7):576–582.

248. Mlyniec K, Davies CL, de Aguero Sanchez IG, Pytka K, Budziszewska B, Nowak G. Essential elements in depression and anxiety. Part I. *Pharmacol. Rep.* 2014;66(4):534–544.

249. Saunders A, Kirk IJ, Waldie KE. Hemispheric coherence in ASD with and without comorbid ADHD and anxiety. *Biomed. Res. Int.* 2016;2016:4267842.

250. Vloet TD, Konrad K, Herpertz-Dahlmann B, Polier GG, Gunther T. Impact of anxiety disorders on attentional functions in children with ADHD. *J. Affect. Disord.* 2010;124(3):283–290.

251. Wilens TE, Kwon A, Tanguay S, et al. Characteristics of adults with attention deficit hyperactivity disorder plus substance use disorder: the role of psychiatric comorbidity. *Am. J. Addict.* 2005;14(4):319–327.

252. Abraham GE. Nutritional factors in the etiology of the premenstrual tension syndromes. *J. Reprod. Med.* 1983;28(7):446–464.

253. Benton D, Donohoe RT. The effects of nutrients on mood. *Public Health Nutr.* 1999;2(3A):403–409.

254. Fathizadeh N, Ebrahimi E, Valiani M, Tavakoli N, Yar MH. Evaluating the effect of magnesium and magnesium plus vitamin B6 supplement on the severity of premenstrual syndrome. *Iran J. Nurs. Midwifery Res.* 2010;15(Suppl 1): 401–405.

255. Spasov AA, Iezhitsa IN, Kharitonova MV, Kravchenko MS. [Depression-like and anxiety-related behaviour of rats fed with magnesium-deficient diet]. *Zh Vyssh Nerv Deiat Im I P Pavlova.* 2008;58(4):476–485.

256. Boyle NB, Lawton CL, Dye L. The effects of magnesium supplementation on subjective anxiety. *Magnes. Res.* 2016;29(3):120–125.

257. Tanabe K, Osada N, Suzuki N, et al. Erythrocyte magnesium and prostaglandin dynamics in chronic sleep deprivation. *Clin. Cardiol.* 1997;20(3):265–268.

258. Alba G, Pereda E, Manas S, et al. The variability of EEG functional connectivity of young ADHD subjects in different resting states. *Clin. Neurophysiol.* 2016;127(2):1321–1330.

chapter ten

Magnesium in obstetrics

David N. Hackney and Alison Bauer

Contents

Introduction

Magnesium sulfate is one of the most commonly administered intravenous medications in pregnancy. The high frequency of usage arises from the fact that it has multiple indications including seizure prophylaxis in a mother with pre-eclampsia and the prevention of cerebral palsy in a fetus that is delivered prematurely. However, the magnitude of supportive evidence varies among the different indications, and the history of magnesium also includes a long period during which it was commonly administered for the prevention of spontaneous preterm birth, despite evidence of non-beneficence.

Physiology

Approximately 40% of magnesium in the human body is protein bound.[1] When magnesium is administered intravenously, it diffuses from the intravascular space to the extravascular space and across the placenta. It will also infuse into uterine muscle (myometrium) tissue.[2] The only portion of magnesium that is measurable by serum concentration is that within the intravascular space, therefore making the volume of distribution difficult to assess. As the magnesium diffuses into the amniotic fluid, there is a delay in the establishment of equilibrium between maternal and fetal plasma, though, with prolonged magnesium administration

135

the magnesium concentration in amniotic fluid is significantly higher than that in maternal plasma.[3] Magnesium is renally excreted during pregnancy. Thus, clinical caution is necessary for pregnant patients with impaired renal function who are also receiving infusions of magnesium.

Pre-eclampsia

Pre-eclampsia is a disease that is unique to pregnant women and remains a mysterious disorder despite significant recent basic science advances. Currently, pre-eclampsia does not have a singular laboratory "gold standard" for diagnosis and is thus clinically defined. The clinical criteria for the diagnosis were reviewed and updated by the American College of Obstetricians and Gynecologists' (ACOG) Task Force on Hypertension in Pregnancy in 2013[4] and is presented in Table 10.1. Diagnostic criteria for the patient without pre-existing chronic hypertension or renal disease includes two elevated blood pressures, > 140 mm Hg systolic or > 90 mm Hg diastolic on two occasions at least 4 hours apart, and proteinuria as defined in Table 10.1. Because pre-eclampsia is clinically defined, a patient will be considered to have the disorder if they meet these criteria, even in the absence of other manifestations. Although it may remain stable for periods of time, the natural history of pre-eclampsia is that it will not

Table 10.1 Diagnostic criteria for pre-eclampsia

Blood pressure	• Systolic blood pressure ≥ 140 mm Hg or diastolic blood pressure ≥ 90 mm Hg on two occasions at least 4 hours apart after 20 weeks of gestation in a woman with previously normal blood pressure • Systolic blood pressure ≥ 160 mm Hg or diastolic blood pressure ≥ 110 mm Hg; hypertension can be confirmed within minutes to facilitate timely treatment with anti-hypertensives
and	
Proteinuria	• ≥ 300 mg of protein in 24-hour urine collection • Or Protein/Creatinine ratio > 0.3 mg/dL • Or Dipstick reading of 1+ (if other quantitative measures are not available)
Or in the absence of proteinuria, new onset hypertension with the new onset of any of the following:	• Thrombocytopenia, platelet count < 100,000/microliter • Renal insufficiency, serum creatinine >1.1 mg/dL or a doubling of serum creatinine in the absence of other renal disease • Impaired liver function, elevated concentrations of liver transaminases to twice normal concentration • Pulmonary edema • Cerebral or visual symptoms

resolve and will eventually worsen prior to delivery. Clinically, patients with pre-eclampsia are divided into those that do or do not have severe manifestations. The ACOG criteria for severe manifestations are outlined in Table 10.2. As is evident from this table, pre-eclampsia can impact a wide range of organ systems including the liver, kidney, and brain. The reason for the diversity of manifestations is that pre-eclampsia fundamentally generates dysfunction of the endothelium[5] by antagonizing vascular endothelial growth factor (VEGF) via placental secretion of the competitive inhibitor soluble fms-like tyrosine kinase (sFLT).[6–8] Endothelial dysfunction, in turn, generates increased extravasation into the extracellular space and subsequent tissue edema which can impact a wide range of human organs. Cerebral edema, for example, accounts for many of the neurologic manifestations of pre-eclampsia, including eclamptic seizures.

Intravenous magnesium has a long history in the management of pre-eclampsia, though it is important to note that it does not treat the underlying disease itself, and delivery of the fetus and placenta remain the only cure. Thus, at its essence, the clinical management of pre-eclampsia entails balancing the severity of an individual patient's disease against the consequences of prematurity at their gestational age and then determining if delivery is appropriate. This is often a difficult decision and the broader clinical management of pre-eclampsia is beyond the scope of this chapter. Intravenous magnesium can, however, prevent seizures in patients with pre-eclampsia. The seizures which can occur because of pre-eclampsia are tonic-clonic in nature and referred to as eclamptic

Table 10.2 Severe features of pre-eclampsia

Severely elevated blood pressure	• Systolic blood pressure ≥ 160 mm Hg or diastolic blood pressure ≥ 110 mm Hg on two occasions at least 4 hours apart while the patient is on bed rest, unless anti-hypertensive therapy is initiated before this time
Thrombocytopenia	• Platelet count < 100,000/microliter
Impaired liver function	• Elevated liver transaminases to twice normal concentration, • Severe, persistent right upper quadrant or epigastric pain, unresponsive to medication and not accounted for by alternative diagnoses, • Or both.
Renal insufficiency	• Serum creatinine concentration > 1.1 mg/dL • Or a doubling of the serum creatinine concentration in the absence of other renal disease.
Pulmonary edema	
New onset cerebral or visual disturbances	

seizures. Likewise, a patient who seizes is then referred to as having eclampsia. Eclampsia has been known since antiquity, though in more modern times it was discovered that many patients experienced blood pressure elevations and proteinuria prior to seizing, and subsequently were identified as being in a state of "pre-eclampsia." These days "pre-eclampsia" is well recognized as a fundamental disorder and impacts around 7% of all pregnant women, very few of whom will ever have an eclamptic seizure. Thus, the disease suffers from unusual semantics in that it continues to be described as "pre-": one of its uncommon terminal manifestations.

Intravenous magnesium is used for both the prevention of initial seizures in patients with pre-eclampsia[9] and recurrent seizures after the first eclamptic event.[10] The mechanism of action, however, continues to be uncertain. Magnesium decreases the vascular tone of placental vessels from pre-eclamptic patients[11] and also lowers endothelin levels.[12] Alternate or contributory mechanisms may also include an inhibition of oxidative damage[13] or cytokine release.[14] Regardless of the exact mechanism, the efficacy for magnesium has been well-demonstrated in large trials.

Between 1998 and 2001, a collaborative group conducted the MAGPIE trial, a randomized placebo-controlled trial evaluating the effectiveness and safety of magnesium sulfate administration for prevention of eclampsia.[9] This study enrolled over 10,000 women at 175 different hospitals throughout 33 different countries. Women were enrolled if they had not yet given birth, or if they were less than 24 hours postpartum, and if they had blood pressure > 140 mm Hg systolic or > 90 mm Hg diastolic on at least two occasions, proteinuria of 1+ or more, and uncertainty whether magnesium sulfate would be clinically beneficial. Their primary outcomes were eclampsia and death of the baby before discharge from the hospital; secondary outcomes included serious maternal morbidity, toxicity, and other side effects of magnesium sulfate administration. Women were randomized to receive either placebo or magnesium sulfate, with a loading dose of 4g and maintenance dose of 1g/hour. This trial found that in women randomized to receive magnesium sulfate, there was no significant difference in maternal mortality, likely because of low maternal mortality rates. However, the relative risk of eclampsia was 58% lower in women randomized to receive magnesium, with a number needed to treat of 63 for women with severe pre-eclampsia and 109 for women without severe pre-eclampsia. For women who were randomized before delivery, there was no significant difference in neonatal death (NNT). The authors found no significant toxicity for mother or baby with magnesium administration. The mode of action of magnesium is unclear, however, they did also find a decrease in the rates of placental abruption for women receiving magnesium, suggesting that magnesium may have beneficial effects on other organ systems affected by pre-eclampsia. This trial was instrumental in demonstrating the reduction in eclampsia with administration of magnesium, as well as the safety of administration without significant toxicity.

Pre-eclampsia is often diagnosed in the antepartum period, however, approximately 5% of women with pre-eclampsia are diagnosed for the first time after delivery, and one-third of eclamptic patients experience their first seizure postpartum.[15] Management of pre-eclampsia in the postpartum period is more clinically unclear. The MAGPIE trial included a subgroup analysis of patients randomized to receive magnesium after delivery and found no statistically significant improvement in neonatal or maternal mortality, or the development of eclampsia with administration of magnesium.[9] Vigil De-Gracia and Ludmir conducted a literature review of the use of magnesium for women with severe pre-eclampsia diagnosed in the postpartum period to further explore this clinical question. They concluded that for women diagnosed with severe pre-eclampsia or eclampsia in the postpartum period, there is no evidence for routine magnesium use as there is little to no effect on the development of seizures with the use of magnesium.

There are multiple dosage regimens for magnesium, including both intravenous and intramuscular regimens, with no clinical consensus on the best route of administration. Salinger et al. conducted a trial in India where they randomized women to receive either intravenous or intramuscular magnesium sulfate regimens, as described in the MAGPIE trial.[16] Women randomized to intravenous administration received a loading dose of 4g over 20 minutes followed by a maintenance dose of 1g/hour. Women randomized to intramuscular administration received a loading dose of 4g intravenously over 20 minutes followed by an intramuscular load of 10 g (5g in each buttock), and a subsequent 5g deep intramuscular dose every 4 hours. They found that the volume of distribution was dependent on maternal weight, with body weight accounting for substantial differences in concentration immediately after the initial bolus was administered. They further found that clearance is inversely dependent on serum creatinine concentration. There is a higher likelihood of developing eclampsia early in the treatment of pre-eclampsia, so obtaining a higher serum concentration early in the course of therapy may be desirable. Minimum therapeutic levels of 4 mEq/L or 4.8 mg/dL have been suggested, however, approximately 25% of women in the intravenous group had serum concentrations <3.5 mg/dL and 25% of women in the intramuscular group had serum concentrations <4.0 mg/dL. Importantly, they concluded that the standard 4g loading dose used in the intravenous regimen results in lower initial concentrations than the intramuscular route. By contrast, using a 6g loading dose with the intravenous regimen would produce similar concentrations to those observed with the intramuscular regimen. They also concluded that serum concentrations are low, and possibly subtherapeutic, in a large proportion of women regardless of the regimen administered; therefore, higher and more personalized dose regimens may be necessary.

As Salinger et al. found, magnesium volume of distribution was closely related to maternal weight. Tudela and colleagues explored the effect of maternal body mass index (BMI) on serum magnesium levels when it was administered for seizure prophylaxis.[17] They proposed that pregnant women with higher BMI would have a higher volume of distribution, which could contribute to subtherapeutic magnesium prophylaxis. This was a retrospective study of over 100,000 patients with severe pre-eclampsia who received magnesium for seizure prophylaxis. The standard regimen used at their institution is a 6g loading dose administered intravenously over 20 minutes, followed by an infusion of 2g per hour. Serum magnesium levels were then obtained 4 hours after treatment was initiated, and levels were considered therapeutic between 4.9–8.4 mg/dL. They found that women classified as obese were significantly more likely to have subtherapeutic magnesium levels, with 61% of obese women presenting with subtherapeutic levels 4 hours after initiation of treatment. When all other risk factors were adjusted for, the odds of a subtherapeutic magnesium level increases with increasing maternal BMI. Therefore, they recommend routine assessment of magnesium levels in obese women with severe pre-eclampsia after initiation of magnesium and to up titration of doses if found to be subtherapeutic.

Neonatal neuroprotection and the prevention of cerebral palsy

Nelson and Grether in 1995[18] identified an epidemiologic association between in utero exposure to magnesium sulfate and a reduced risk of cerebral palsy, a finding that was corroborated in some[19] though not all[20] follow up studies. Similar to the reduction in maternal seizure risk among patients with pre-eclampsia, the exact mechanism of neuroprotection in the fetus and neonate remains uncertain. One contributing factor may be a reduction in cytokine expression[14, 21, 22] and in animal test subjects magnesium is able to reduce neural injury secondary to exposure to lipopolysaccharide.[23] An alternate or contributory mechanism could also be a resistance to ischemia or injury via an inhibition of excitatory amino acids, particularly N-methyl-D-aspartate (NMDA).[24] Magnesium may also decrease the blood-brain barrier permeability.[25]

Regardless of the exact mechanism, the utility of magnesium for cerebral palsy prior to preterm birth is now well established. Specifically, three large multicenter randomized trials[26–28] were conducted in the United States, Australia, and France which enrolled pregnant women delivering prematurely prior to gestational ages ranging from 30 to 33 weeks. All studies also included multiyear follow-up. Although exact findings and outcomes varied between trials, a reduction in cerebral palsy has been demonstrated in meta-analysis.[29] Thus, intravenous magnesium infusion is now recommended prior to preterm delivery by the ACOG.[30] Of note, although the reduction in cerebral palsy is statistically significant, the total magnitude of the risk reduction is small, with an estimated number needed to treat (NNT) of 63.[29] Also, pre-delivery magnesium does not appear to reduce the risk of mortality or other outcomes. Despite the small magnitude of benefit, however, most patients can receive intravenous magnesium safely with a relatively low incidence of serious side effects. Additionally, because cerebral palsy is a life-long and potentially debilitating disorder, even a small reduction is potentially tremendously beneficial. Likewise, cost-effectiveness analysis has still favored magnesium administration prior to preterm birth.[31]

Tocolysis

In addition to its well-validated use in fetal neuroprotection and maternal seizure prophylaxis, there is also a long history of magnesium being used to prevent delivery in patients experiencing spontaneous preterm labor. Unfortunately, the preponderance of clinical evidence does not support this practice and it is no longer recommended by most experts.[32] Medications that decrease uterine contractions in preterm labor are referred to as tocolytics. The ideal tocolytic agent would target the central predominantly smooth muscle portion of the uterus known as the myometrium while sparing smooth and striated muscles in other locations in the body. Tocolytics are used in the hope that by suppressing uterine activity in preterm labor one can prevent or delay the delivery of the fetus, and thus improve the neonatal outcomes. On its surface, this is a logical therapeutic approach, though as is often the case in medicine, clinical trials have yielded a more complicated picture. Specifically, the administration of any tocolytic agent has never been demonstrated to improve neonatal clinical outcomes even with medications that, unlike magnesium, actually successfully delay preterm birth by 48 hours or longer.[33] Thus, it is unclear in the first place if neonatal outcomes can be improved by preventing preterm birth after the initiation of spontaneous labor. The reasons for this remain unclear and include the possibility that a true benefit to tocolysis does exist, but has not yet been identified secondary to the design and statistical power of the existing trials. Another possibility, however, is that the artificial maintenance of the fetus in the uterus in the context of spontaneous preterm labor is actually harmful. The instigators of preterm labor include intrauterine infections and inflammation as well as placental bleeding events, many of which may not be clinically evident and thus known to the obstetrician at the time of preterm labor. Thus, using medications to artificially prevent delivery in these contexts may prolong fetal exposure to infectious agents, inflammation, or other adverse events; the harm of which may outweigh the benefits of delaying preterm birth.

Regardless of the larger question of whether or not tocolysis is beneficial, intravenous magnesium is not itself a tocolytic in that it does not alter term or preterm labor in any meaningful clinical context. This is somewhat counterintuitive with regards to the known understanding of myometrial contractility and available in vitro studies. Like all smooth muscles, myometrial contractions are triggered by an increase in intracellular calcium which in turn activates myosin light chain kinase (MLKC). MLKC, in turn, phosphorylates myosin leading to its activation and interaction with actin which ultimately generates the contraction of the entire muscle cell. Thus, one could inhibit myometrial contractions by antagonizing calcium on a cellular level, and likewise, one of the other commonly used categories of tocolytic agents are calcium channel blockers (CCB), such as nifedipine.[34] Likewise, in vitro myometrial samples exposed to high concentrations of magnesium will demonstrate impaired contractility in conjunction with decreased intracellular concentrations of calcium.[35]

Thus, the original belief that magnesium could be a tocolytic agent was grounded in biologic plausibility. Additionally, many patients who present in acute preterm labor are observed to stop contracting, and subsequently continue their pregnancies undelivered, after the intravenous administration of magnesium. This combination of biologic plausibility and clinical observation led many experts to recommend intravenous magnesium infusions in the treatment of patients experiencing acute preterm labor, and magnesium tocolysis subsequently became widely adopted clinically. Multiple controlled clinical trials, however, have not supported this practice. Most fundamentally, intravenous magnesium failed to prolong pregnancy or prevent preterm delivery when compared to placebo or no treatment in randomized controlled trials[36–39] as well as meta-analyses of the combined trials results.[40] Several more indirect lines of evidence also support the results of the controlled clinical trials. For example, a dose-response relationship should exist for any truly efficacious therapeutic agent such that the magnitude of the clinical response increases with the administered dose or serum concentration. However, there has been no demonstrable association between uterine contraction frequency and serum magnesium concentrations in patients undergoing magnesium tocolysis.[41] Additionally, intravenous magnesium has not been demonstrated to impact labor characteristics when studied in contexts other than tocolysis. For example, when patients in term labor received magnesium for seizure prophylaxis in pre-eclampsia there were no differences in the length between those who did or did not receive magnesium.[42,43] Likewise, no differences in latency after preterm membrane rupture was identified among patients who did or did not receive intravenous magnesium for neuroprotection.[44]

Why does the intravenous administration of magnesium not impact term or preterm labor despite being a calcium antagonist? The answer is likely that increasing magnesium serum concentrations is not in any way specific to the uterine myometrium and thus, clinically meaningful reductions in uterine contractions cannot be obtained without broader muscular inhibitions and thus toxicity. Likewise, one of the contemporaneous categories of tocolytic agents is oxytocin-receptor antagonists[45] which are obviously much more specific to the myometrium. However, if intravenous magnesium does not inhibit labor, then what would explain the clinical observation that many women in spontaneous preterm labor stop contracting and their pregnancies remain undelivered after receiving it? The answer is that, for reasons that are incompletely understood, many patients who present in spontaneous preterm labor will stop contracting and their pregnancies remain undelivered even with no treatment or the administration of a placebo. In a systematic review of all published subjects with spontaneous preterm labor who did not receive tocolysis, a majority (62.8%) remained undelivered at 48 hours and 40.4% actually still delivered at term.[46] Explanations for these observations include the fact that preterm labor remains clinically, and thus imperfectly, diagnosed. Even for patients in "true" preterm labor, however, the progression to delivery may not be as linear or uniform as one may intuitively believe.

Despite the shift away from magnesium for tocolysis most patients delivering prematurely do and should still receive magnesium albeit for the validated indication of fetal neuroprotection and the prevention of cerebral palsy as described previously. Although superficially both tocolysis and neuroprotection may involve intravenously administering magnesium to patients in spontaneous preterm labor, there are important practical differences. Specifically, for fetal neuroprotection to be impactful, the magnesium needs to be infused at the time of delivery itself so that the fetal neurologic magnesium concentrations are increased when first extra-uterine. However, when magnesium was previously used as a tocolytic, though not neuroprotection, it was used early in the labor process in an attempt to arrest the contractions, though it was usually discontinued before delivery. This is because tocolysis is generally discontinued secondary to perceived futility if labor progresses despite the tocolytic, and delivery becomes inevitable. On the other hand, if a patient is in early spontaneous preterm labor though still temporally remote from delivery itself, there is no clear role for magnesium neuroprotection at that time, and magnesium would not be indicated for the preterm labor alone. Finally, if a patient in spontaneous preterm labor is receiving magnesium for fetal neuroprotection and it is clinically determined that tocolysis would be appropriate, consideration would need to be given to the additional administration of a medication with known tocolytic efficacy as the magnesium itself would not be beneficial in this regard. In combination, the historic use of magnesium for tocolysis was unfortunate because it occurred in the absence of supportive clinical trial data, potentially precluded the use of more efficacious tocolytic agents, and exposed patients to unnecessary magnesium side effects and possible toxicity.

Magnesium toxicity

While magnesium is being administered, patients should be monitored closely for adverse effects and signs of toxicity, including assessment of respiratory rate, patellar reflexes, neurologic status, and urine output. Since magnesium is cleared renally, if significant oliguria is present, the patient is at risk for toxicity and providers should consider holding the magnesium dose until urine output improves.

Smith and colleagues[47] performed an integrative review of 54 clinical studies, including 9556 women who received magnesium to explore the side effects related to magnesium administration. The overall incidence of absent patellar reflex was 1.6%, of respiratory depression was 1.3%, of the need for calcium gluconate was 0.2%, and only one maternal death was attributed by the authors to use of magnesium. The maternal death was secondary to respiratory depression, and her serum magnesium level was supratherapeutic at 24 mEq/L.

Adverse effects of magnesium, which can occur at plasma concentrations of 3.8-5 mmol/L, include flushing, headaches, blurred vision, nausea and vomiting, nystagmus, lethargy, hypothermia, urinary retention, fecal impaction, muscle weakness, dizziness, and irritation at the injection.

At plasma concentrations of 3.5-5 mmol/L, the patellar reflex may decrease, and loss of the patellar reflex is the first warning sign for impending toxicity. At therapeutic levels of magnesium, reflexes may be decreased but will remain present. If reflexes are present, plasma magnesium concentration is rarely toxic. However, at plasma concentrations of 5-6.5 mmol/L, respiratory paralysis may occur, at plasma concentrations greater than 7.5 mmol/L, cardiac conduction is altered, and at plasma concentrations greater than 12.5 mmol/L, cardiac arrest can occur. Magnesium also readily crosses the placenta, and infants exposed to magnesium may experience respiratory depression and hyporeflexia.

Greenberg et al. conducted a retrospective cohort study and explored the effects of magnesium sulfate administration on term neonates born to mothers with pre-eclampsia.[48] All included children were >37 weeks, single gestation, born to women with pre-eclampsia, who either did or did not receive magnesium for seizure prophylaxis prior to delivery. Their primary outcome was admission to the neonatal intensive care unit. Infants exposed to magnesium sulfate were significantly more likely to require admission to the neonatal intensive care unit, with a number needed to harm (NNH) of 11. When the authors performed a multivariable regression, magnesium sulfate exposure was still significantly associated with an increased likelihood for admission to the neonatal intensive care unit, with an adjusted odds ratio of 3.69. The likelihood of admission to the neonatal intensive care unit further increased with prolonged magnesium sulfate exposure. For infants who were exposed to magnesium sulfate for >12 hours compared to infants exposed <12 hours, the number needed to harm with magnesium sulfate exposure >12 hours was 5 and with exposure <12 hours was 7. They concluded that there is a dose-response association between antenatal magnesium sulfate exposure and neonatal intensive care unit admission, likely related to the magnesium sulfate leading to depressed neonatal and gastrointestinal tone. They concluded that given the increased needs of infants exposed to magnesium sulfate and the low number needed to harm, all neonates exposed to magnesium sulfate in the immediate antenatal period should be routinely assessed for possible increased care requirements.

Conclusions

Intravenous magnesium has a long and complicated history of clinical use in obstetrics. Its predominant role is in neuronal stabilization and the prevention of neurologic injury including both eclamptic seizures in the mother and cerebral palsy after preterm delivery in the neonate. Although administered to many patients in spontaneous preterm labor for fetal neuroprotection, magnesium is not contemporaneously considered to be a tocolytic or to otherwise impact the course of term or preterm labor itself. Mild side effects are common with intravenous administration and all patients receiving magnesium also need to undergo close monitoring for more severe toxicity. With proper clinical use, however, magnesium provides important benefits to many women facing serious complications in their pregnancies.

References

1. Lu, J.F. and C.H. Nightingale, Magnesium sulfate in eclampsia and pre-eclampsia: pharmacokinetic principles. *Clin Pharmacokinet*, 2000. 38(4): p. 305–14.
2. Lemancewicz, A., et al., Permeability of fetal membranes to calcium and magnesium: possible role in preterm labour. *Hum Reprod*, 2000. 15(9): p. 2018–22.
3. Hallak, M., et al., Fetal serum and amniotic fluid magnesium concentrations with maternal treatment. *Obstet Gynecol*, 1993. 81(2): p. 185–8.

4. Hypertension in pregnancy. Report of the American College of Obstetricians and Gynecologists' Task Force on Hypertension in Pregnancy. *Obstet Gynecol*, 2013. 122(5): p. 1122–31.
5. Roberts, J.M., et al., Preeclampsia: an endothelial cell disorder. *Am J Obstet Gynecol*, 1989. 161(5): p. 1200–4.
6. Levine, R.J., et al., Circulating angiogenic factors and the risk of preeclampsia. *N Engl J Med*, 2004. 350(7): p. 672–83.
7. McKeeman, G.C., et al., Soluble vascular endothelial growth factor receptor-1 (sFlt-1) is increased throughout gestation in patients who have preeclampsia develop. *Am J Obstet Gynecol*, 2004. 191(4): p. 1240–6.
8. Nagamatsu, T., et al., Cytotrophoblasts up-regulate soluble fms-like tyrosine kinase-1 expression under reduced oxygen: an implication for the placental vascular development and the pathophysiology of preeclampsia. *Endocrinology*, 2004. 145(11): p. 4838–45.
9. Altman, D., et al., Do women with pre-eclampsia, and their babies, benefit from magnesium sulphate? The Magpie Trial: a randomised placebo-controlled trial. *Lancet*, 2002. 359(9321): p. 1877–90.
10. Which anticonvulsant for women with eclampsia? Evidence from the Collaborative Eclampsia Trial. *Lancet*, 1995. 345(8963): p. 1455–63.
11. Kovac, C.M., et al., Fetoplacental vascular tone is modified by magnesium sulfate in the preeclamptic ex vivo human placental cotyledon. *Am J Obstet Gynecol*, 2003. 189(3): p. 839–42.
12. Mastrogiannis, D.S., et al., Effect of magnesium sulfate on plasma endothelin-1 levels in normal and preeclamptic pregnancies.*Am J Obstet Gynecol*, 1992. 167(6): p. 1554–9.
13. Abad, C., et al., Magnesium sulfate affords protection against oxidative damage during severe preeclampsia. *Placenta*, 2015. 36(2): p. 179–85.
14. Blackwell, S.C., et al., The effects of intrapartum magnesium sulfate therapy on fetal serum interleukin-1beta, interleukin-6, and tumor necrosis factor-alpha at delivery: a randomized, placebo-controlled trial. *Am J Obstet Gynecol*, 2001. 184(7): p. 1320–3; discussion 1323–4.
15. Vigil-De Gracia, P. and J. Ludmir, The use of magnesium sulfate for women with severe preeclampsia or eclampsia diagnosed during the postpartum period. *J Matern Fetal Neonatal Med*, 2015. 28(18): p. 2207–9.
16. Salinger, D.H., et al., Magnesium sulphate for prevention of eclampsia: are intramuscular and intravenous regimens equivalent? A population pharmacokinetic study. *Bjog*, 2013. 120(7): p. 894–900.
17. Tudela, C.M., D.D. McIntire, and J.M. Alexander, Effect of maternal body mass index on serum magnesium levels given for seizure prophylaxis. *Obstet Gynecol*, 2013. 121(2 Pt 1): p. 314–20.
18. Nelson, K.B. and J.K. Grether, Can magnesium sulfate reduce the risk of cerebral palsy in very low birthweight infants? *Pediatrics*, 1995. 95(2): p. 263–9.
19. Schendel, D.E., et al., Prenatal magnesium sulfate exposure and the risk for cerebral palsy or mental retardation among very low-birth-weight children aged 3 to 5 years. *JAMA*, 1996. 276(22): p. 1805–10.
20. Paneth, N., et al., Magnesium sulfate in labor and risk of neonatal brain lesions and cerebral palsy in low birth weight infants. The Neonatal Brain Hemorrhage Study Analysis Group. *Pediatrics*, 1997. 99(5): p. E1.

21. Suzuki-Kakisaka, H., et al., Magnesium sulfate increases intracellular magnesium reducing inflammatory cytokine release in neonates. *Am J Reprod Immunol*, 2013. 70(3): p. 213–20.

22. Sugimoto, J., et al., Magnesium decreases inflammatory cytokine production: a novel innate immunomodulatory mechanism. *J Immunol*, 2012. 188(12): p. 6338–46.

23. Burd, I., et al., Magnesium sulfate reduces inflammation-associated brain injury in fetal mice. *Am JObstet Gynecol*, 2010. 202(3): p. 292.e1–9.

24. McDonald, J.W., F.S. Silverstein, and M.V. Johnston, Magnesium reduces N-methyl-D-aspartate (NMDA)-mediated brain injury in perinatal rats. *Neurosci Lett*, 1990. 109(1–2): p. 234–8.

25. Kaya, M., et al., Magnesium sulfate attenuates increased blood-brain barrier permeability during insulin-induced hypoglycemia in rats. *Can J Physiol Pharmacol*, 2001. 79(9): p. 793–8.

26. Rouse, D.J., et al., A randomized, controlled trial of magnesium sulfate for the prevention of cerebral palsy. *N Engl J Med*, 2008. 359(9): p. 895–905.

27. Crowther, C.A., et al., Effect of magnesium sulfate given for neuroprotection before preterm birth: a randomized controlled trial. *JAMA*, 2003. 290(20): p. 2669–76.

28. Marret, S., et al., [Effect of magnesium sulphate on mortality and neurologic morbidity of the very-preterm newborn (of less than 33 weeks) with two-year neurological outcome: results of the prospective PREMAG trial]. *Gynecol Obstet Fertil*, 2008. 36(3): p. 278–88.

29. Costantine, M.M. and S.J. Weiner, Effects of antenatal exposure to magnesium sulfate on neuroprotection and mortality in preterm infants: a meta-analysis. *Obstet Gynecol*, 2009. 114(2 Pt 1): p. 354–64.

30. Committee Opinion No. 455: Magnesium sulfate before anticipated preterm birth for neuroprotection. *Obstet Gynecol*, 2010. 115(3): p. 669–71.

31. Cahill, A.G., et al., Magnesium sulfate therapy for the prevention of cerebral palsy in preterm infants: a decision-analytic and economic analysis. *Am J Obstet Gynecol*, 2011. 205(6): p. 542.e1–7.

32. Grimes, D.A. and K. Nanda, Magnesium sulfate tocolysis: time to quit. *Obstet Gynecol*, 2006. 108(4): p. 986–9.

33. Gyetvai, K., et al., Tocolytics for preterm labor: a systematic review. *Obstet Gynecol*, 1999. 94(5 Pt 2): p. 869–77.

34. Flenady, V., et al., Calcium channel blockers for inhibiting preterm labour and birth. *Cochrane Database Syst Rev*, 2014. (6): p. Cd002255.

35. Fomin, V.P., et al., Effect of magnesium sulfate on contractile force and intracellular calcium concentration in pregnant human myometrium. *Am J Obstet Gynecol*, 2006. 194(5): p. 1384–90.

36. Fox, M.D., et al., Neonatal morbidity between 34 and 37 weeks' gestation. *J Perinatol*, 1993. 13(5): p. 349–53.

37. How, H.Y., et al., Tocolysis in women with preterm labor between 32 0/7 and 34 6/7 weeks of gestation: a randomized controlled pilot study. *Am J Obstet Gynecol*, 2006. 194(4): p. 976–81.

38. Cotton, D.B., et al., Comparison of magnesium sulfate, terbutaline and a placebo for inhibition of preterm labor. A randomized study. *J Reprod Med*, 1984. 29(2): p. 92–7.

39. Cox, S.M., M.L. Sherman, and K.J. Leveno, Randomized investigation of magnesium sulfate for prevention of preterm birth. *Am J Obstet Gynecol*, 1990. 163(3): p. 767–72.

40. Crowther, C.A., et al., Magnesium sulphate for preventing preterm birth in threatened preterm labour. *Cochrane Database Syst Rev*, 2014. (8): p. Cd001060.

41. Madden, C., J. Owen, and J.C. Hauth, Magnesium tocolysis: serum levels versus success. *Am J Obstet Gynecol*, 1990. 162(5): p. 1177–80.

42. Szal, S.E., M.S. Croughan-Minihane, and S.J. Kilpatrick, Effect of magnesium prophylaxis and preeclampsia on the duration of labor. *Am J Obstet Gynecol*, 1999. 180(6 Pt 1): p. 1475–9.

43. Witlin, A.G., S.A. Friedman, and B.M. Sibai, The effect of magnesium sulfate therapy on the duration of labor in women with mild preeclampsia at term: a randomized, double-blind, placebo-controlled trial. *Am J Obstet Gynecol*, 1997. 176(3): p. 623–7.

44. Horton, A.L., et al., Effect of magnesium sulfate administration for neuro-protection on latency in women with preterm premature rupture of membranes. *Am J Perinatol*, 2015. 32(4): p. 387–92.

45. Flenady, V., et al., Oxytocin receptor antagonists for inhibiting preterm labour. *Cochrane Database Syst Rev*, 2014. (6): p. Cd004452.

46. Hackney, D.N., C. Olson-Chen, and L.L. Thornburg, What do we know about the natural outcomes of preterm labour? A systematic review and meta-analysis of women without tocolysis in preterm labour. *Paediatr Perinat Epidemiol*, 2013. 27(5): p. 452–60.

47. Smith, J.M., et al., An integrative review of the side effects related to the use of magnesium sulfate for pre-eclampsia and eclampsia management. *BMC Pregnancy Childbirth*, 2013. 13: p. 34.

48. Greenberg, M.B., et al., Effect of magnesium sulfate exposure on term neo-nates. *J Perinatol*, 2013. 33(3): p. 188–93.

Index